Attending
Children

a doctor's education

M ARGARET E. M OHRMANN

GEORGETOWN UNIVERSITY PRESS
Washington, D.C.

As of January 1, 2007, 13-digit ISBN numbers will replace the current 10-digit system.
Cloth: 978-1-58901-054-3
Paperback: 978-1-58901-107-6

First Georgetown University Press paperback edition, 2006
ISBN 1-58901-107-4 (paper : alk. paper)

Georgetown University Press, Washington, D.C.

This book is printed on acid-free paper meeting the requirements of the American
National Standard for Permanence in Paper for Printed Library Materials.

Library of Congress Cataloging-in-Publication Data

Mohrmann, Margaret E., 1948–
    Attending children : a doctor's education / Margaret E. Mohrmann.
        p.   cm.
    Includes biographical references.
    ISBN 1-58901-054-X (cloth : alk. paper)
    1. Mohrmann, Margaret E., 1948–   2. Pediatricians—Biography.
    3. Pediatrics—Study and teaching (Internship)   4. Physician and patient.
    [DNLM: I. Mohrmann, Margaret E., 1948–   2. Pediatrics–Personal
    Narratives.   3. Education, Medical.   4. Patients.   5. Physician-Patient
    Relations—Personal Narratives. WZ 100 M6993 2005]   I.   Title.
    RJ43.M64A3   2005
    618.92'00092—dc22   2004023156

13 12 11 10 09 08 07 06   9 8 7 6 5 4 3 2
First printing

Printed in the United States of America

In memory and in honor of
the children and parents who taught me my vocation,
this book has been written with gratitude, humility, and love.
In particular, I remember
Margaret Mary (Mickey) Madary,
January 25, 1962–November 20, 1974.

These days, doctors are encouraged to shovel everything into a computer, for the sake of epidemiology, statistics, accountants. But no one seems interested in etching the names and faces of people into memory, or recalling the first encounter, the early feelings, the surprises, the comic details, the tragic stories, the failures of understanding, the silences. I've seen thousands of people go by, but at this exact moment I couldn't readily call up more than a dozen of them—twenty with some time, maybe fifty if I strained a little, but not many more. . . .

So, I think that writing, for a doctor like for anyone else, is a way to take the measure of what we don't remember, what we don't retain. You write to try to knit up the holes in evanescent reality with bits of string, tie knots in transparent veils, knowing that they're going to tear open somewhere else. One writes against memory, not with it.

One writes to measure loss.

—Martin Winckler, *The Case of Doctor Sachs*

Contents

Acknowledgments

A FEW YEARS AGO, Richard Brown, director of the Georgetown University Press and friend of many years, proposed that I write a book of stories from my career as a pediatrician. I had not considered such a project before, and the idea took quite a bit of pondering before I decided to do it. It would not have happened without his suggestion, and now, having done it, I know it was a very good thing to do—for me, without question, and I hope also for my readers. Furthermore, it is a much better book because of his gentle and perceptive editing skills. My first and fervent thanks go to Richard, best of editors, excellent friend.

The University of Virginia generously granted my request for a half-year leave during which to write the book. I am grateful to the Program of Humanities in Medicine and the Department of Religious Studies for allowing me time away from teaching and administrative responsibilities to devote to this task.

The list of people whose contributions to this work should be acknowledged is virtually limitless. These stories cover thirty years of my adult life, during which so many people have touched, guided, inspired, and challenged me. An enumeration would begin with my ever-supportive and deeply loving parents and include my many teachers, in all their guises; nurses, without whom I could never have learned how to be a doctor; physician colleagues, who provided so many good, and a few instructively bad, models of conscientious doctoring; students and residents, for whom I had to find a way not only to show but also to say what I know; church communities and friends, who helped create and faithfully sustained the inner resources I could bring to the work; and, of course, the patients and their families who consistently gave me, along with so much else, the immeasurable privilege of being their doctor.

There are, however, some persons who deserve particular mention. You will meet those who were patients and family members of patients in the following stories, which I have written in constant awareness of the debt of gratitude and fidelity I owe them all. Specifically, I thank Marshall and Mary Madary, Tony Leaphart, and Vonnie Yarborough Leaphart for giving me permission not only to tell the story of this part of their lives but also to use their names in doing so. I can only begin, with this offering of remembrance and love, to thank them for welcoming me into their lives beyond my care of their children so many years ago.

Nurses have played a most important role in my life as a physician, teaching me so much of my craft, showing me how much more there is to patient care than technical know-how. Among the nurses who have changed my life, no one is more important than Jane Lunn, who was the head nurse of the pediatric intensive care unit I directed in the 1980s. Our close and enduring friendship was forged in the shared experiences of that time. Jane was a participant in most of the stories I recount in part II; directly or indirectly, she has been part of all the various aspects of my career and my life over the last twenty-plus years. Not only is she my primary model of an excellent nurse, but she is also indispensable as an honest sounding board, auxiliary conscience, loyal advocate, and boon companion.

Several months before I began writing this book, I participated in the annual summer seminar at Hiram College, led by Carol Donley and Martin Kohn, directors of the college's Center for Literature, Medicine, and the Health Professions. The entire weeklong course was renewing, illuminating, and invigorating, but I am especially grateful for the group's discussing with me the ethics of writing stories about patients and helping me to consider more deeply the nature of the mutual trust involved in the physician-patient interaction that forms the story and to recognize the stories as also mine, integral parts of my own life. Later discussion with Anne Hunsaker Hawkins, augmented by her essay (written with Jack Coulehan and referred to in the Introduction), was also invaluable for my working through these matters of confidentiality, privacy, and "ownership."

I am particularly indebted to colleagues and friends who read the book in draft form and offered immensely helpful observations, corrections, and suggestions for improvement, as well as enthusiastic support for the project. Larry Bouchard, Marcia Day Childress, Anne Hawkins, Aline Kalbian, and Vanessa Ochs each pushed me to think—and write—more clearly about certain aspects of what I was doing and, as a result, have made the book much better than it would have been. Responsibility for the remaining flaws is entirely my own.

There can be few joys to equal having, as I do, a life partner who knows firsthand the sorts of experiences a career in medicine affords and shares my perspective on them. Deborah Healey has been my cocreator in this work, affirming the importance of telling the stories, sharing memories of her own years as a resident and then practitioner of pediatrics, as well as newer insights and experiences gleaned from her retraining as a psychiatrist. She has corroborated, amended, and expanded my understanding of doctoring while serving—with sustained interest through numerous drafts—as my most rigorous critic and editor. Although the words are hopelessly inadequate, I am grateful *to* her for her unflagging willingness to be part of the adventure of writing this book, as I am grateful each day *for* her and our life together.

Introduction: Attending

Attend: from the Latin *ad tendere*: to stretch to or toward

THIS IS A BOOK of stories from my career as a pediatrician in academic medical centers. These stories are the episodes that have formed my understanding of medical practice by revealing the nature of the suffering that presents itself to medicine, the resources upon which people—doctors as well as patients—draw when confronted by such suffering, the questions that recur, the tasks of medical education, and the obligations, powers, and privileges of the physician. More than that, these are the stories that have formed *me*, as a doctor, a teacher, a theological ethicist, and a person.

Why write them for others to read? Surely part of the reason is encapsulated in the words of physician Marc Zaffran (writing as Martin Winckler) in the epigraph of this book: to inscribe names and faces, to measure what is lost, to tie up the holes in what remains—to hold on to what I know and try to make sense of it as a whole. Beyond the need to shore up my own understandings, however, I wish with these stories to display and argue for the central significance of such experiences in the intellectual and spiritual formation of physicians.

Arthur Frank, in *The Wounded Storyteller*, encourages those who would reflect on and write about illness, healing, and the ethics of medicine to think *with* stories. As he explains,

> To think about a story is to reduce it to content and then analyze that content. Thinking with stories takes the story as already complete; there is no going beyond it. To think with a story is to experience it affecting one's own life and to find in that effect a certain truth of one's life. . . . Thinking with stories ultimately requires a highly personal sedimentation of experience: living with the stories and having them shape perceptions of various experiences over time.[1]

With this book I respond to Frank's welcome challenge by presenting stories of children and their parents in their encounter with medicine and, consequently, with me. I submit the stories as "already complete," at least in the sense I believe Frank intends: without significant embellishment or interpretation, despite occasional reflective asides. They are, of course, manifestly *in*complete. I am not an omniscient narrator. I have done the best I can to reconstruct the encounters from what I remember, but memory, notoriously selective, has its own untraceable editing hand. Besides, like all stories, these tales can be only fragments of the life narratives they recount.

I offer these stories for the express purpose of thinking with them about the profession and practice of medicine and, more specifically, about a crucial part of medical education: how doctors learn to *be* doctors—that is, how physicians learn to attend to patients, as opposed to how they learn scientific facts of human physiology and disease. Rather than compose a treatise on this subject, which has become a central focus of my professional work, I ponder and present the topic through the medium of narrative. In doing so, I express my convictions about the preeminent value of this medium for revealing what physicians are called—morally, intellectually, and emotionally—to be and to do by the patients who are their life's work.

Therefore, this book is inevitably "a highly personal sedimentation of experience." I started this project with the desire to give these children I have cared for (in both senses of that phrase) the voices they did not and do not have. Sick persons and children are two of several voiceless segments of our society—sick children are doubly mute. There have been a number of collections of "doctor stories" published in recent years, but too often these can appear to exploit the experiences of particular patients in order to highlight the skills of the doctor, trumpet the triumphs of American medicine, or trade on the public's appetite for gee-whiz tales of adventure and derring-do in the emergency room, the operating suite, or the front lines of epidemic warfare. I wanted my collection of stories to be something different: not the stentorian claims of medicine and its practitioners, but the voices—whatever their timbre or volume—of children and their parents, who have found themselves unwillingly cast in the role of patients in medicine's theater. I wish to honor the truth of their lives and sufferings, both in gratitude for what they have given me by allowing me a part in their drama and in the conviction that their lives and deaths matter and are worth reporting.

But this issue of voice is complicated. The voice you will hear in these stories is, of course, mine. Not only am I telling patients' stories second-hand, as it were, mediating and translating their voices, but also I am able to tell only those parts of their narratives that also included me. There seems to be no way around the basic problem of the medical voice co-opting the patient's story. Mine is inescapably a medical voice; I can speak of these patients only because I knew them as their doctor. Even with this proviso, however, I can assert that these are not case narratives of the usual sort found in texts and journals of medicine or bioethics. Rather, they are accounts of the intersections of the lives of specific children and their families with my life, intersections occasioned by the professional connection. They are a reflection of life at those crossings only, but life as it happens, nevertheless.[2]

Anne Hunsaker Hawkins, whose masterly writing about narrative in ethics and medicine has been a touchstone for me, writes,

> We should remember that every ethical decision marks the intersection of two life stories, the patient's and the physician's, and epiphanic moments of imaginative insight or intuitive understanding occur in both. These are the lyric moments in the prose of our everyday experience.[3]

Everything about a medical encounter represents a junction of at least two life stories. If I am to think with stories, I have only the narratives of life at this crossroads, where my work as a doctor and the exigencies of my patients' situations meet and give rise to the lyric moments that I articulate in this book.

So, the voice is mine, and it changes, as I do, over the chronologically ordered course of these stories. I have tried to be faithful both to who I was at each encounter and, especially, to the experiences of the children and parents I met and lived with for a time. The stories are as thorough as I can make them. Sometimes my relationship with a patient lasted days, sometimes years. Some children I knew only during their brief time in the pediatric intensive care unit; some I followed from childhood through adolescence.

These stories are true, although not absolutely factual. Of the nineteen narratives included in these fourteen chapters, there are two (Mickey's story in chapter 4 and Lindsey's in chapter 9) for which I have requested and received, from the parents of each child, permission to use real names and descriptions. For most of the other stories, it has not been possible for me to locate the now-grown children or their surviving families to ask permission. The majority of these encounters happened twenty years ago or more. Families have moved on; I have forgotten last names. I have no standing in the medical centers where I used to work that would allow me to explore old records in a search for names and addresses. Even some of the more recent patients and families have proven to be unreachable. There are also a few stories told here of children and parents whom I may have been able to contact, had I tried; I chose not to do so because I did not believe it would be in their best interests, but felt strongly that the disguised story should be told nonetheless.

The preceding paragraph summarizes the result of my protracted wrestling with questions of consent, confidentiality, and privacy. I have tried to focus on finding and maintaining a proper balance between, on the one hand, my moral obligation to keep my patients from being harmed in any way by their relationship with me and, on the other, my moral obligation to participate meaningfully in the edification not only of medical students and physicians but also of medicine's observers, critics, and consumers, its once and future patients. That is, I have tried to be truthful—to present the realities of some people's encounters with illness and of what doctors may be called upon to do and to be—without scattering abroad facts that should remain private.[4]

I have intentionally changed not only names but also varying combinations of characteristics—age, diagnosis, physical description, gender, parental occupation—when doing so did not seem to alter substantially the weight and direction of the narrative. In the two chapters in which I have family permission to use real names and circumstances, I have changed information about ancillary characters, such as other physicians, nurses, and social workers. Undoubtedly, many other details have been altered unintentionally by the vagaries of memory. These are the stories as I remember them, seasoned by years, even decades, of turning them over in my mind, rubbing them like talismans for luck and wisdom until they glow—and all I can see of them now are the parts that shine.

Almost thirty years after I began my career in medicine, I stopped practicing pediatrics. My vocational attention had been drawn to teaching and writing at the intersection of medicine, religion, and ethics, and I was no longer able, or willing, to devote enough hours to the clinic to sustain a primary care practice. The transition was gradual; I decreased my practice time over several years, so the ending was not too abrupt—for me. For some of my patients, my departure may have seemed both sudden and puzzling. A few parents who had come to know me well smiled at the news and said they had always known that teaching was my first love. Others perhaps thought what Mrs. Morris (chapter 13) wrote: "You don't want to be a doctor."

But that statement would be incorrect. It is not a matter of whether I want to be a doctor. I *am* a doctor, whether I practice medicine or not. The years of medical school and residency, of attending to acutely and chronically ill children, of teaching and rounding with students and residents, of following children in the clinic, of conferring with parents, colleagues, and consultants—those years molded me as surely as a career in the military must permanently stiffen one's spine. Whatever activity I engage in, my posture is that of a physician, shaped by countless patients and parents who have bent my ear, reached for my hand, touched my heart.

Sometimes I think that I had to stop practicing because I had been filled to overflowing. Not burned out—that is not how it has ever felt—but impatient to pour out what I had learned into some articulation of its significance for educating doctors and for understanding what medicine is at its core, to explore or even create paths of interconnection between the practical truths of the lives and deaths I have known and the speculative wisdoms of theology, history, literature, and ethics.

⅍ Exemplary Stories

THE STORIES in this book are selected from among the thousands of patient encounters I had through thirty years in pediatrics. Why these?

They are, for one reason or another, tales that live in my mind. I kept no journal notes, no files of "interesting" or moving case reports. These are the children I have never forgotten, the ones whose names became shorthand tags for milestones along my never-ending path of initiation into the art of doctoring. Although most of the names have been changed for this book, the real names are as clear and present to me as the names of persons in my family. Their stories have come back to me, usually unbidden, over and over, coaching me as I attended to new patients and their parents, suggesting what needed to be said to a student or a resident, telling me who I am and where I am headed within this profession. Some serve as guides and reminders, others as warnings and brakes. However, they are not so much metaphorical signposts and traffic signals as they are, taken together, the embodiment and most authentic expression of my understanding of the depth and preciousness of doctoring and the courage and fragility of children and families in crisis.

To Wittgenstein is attributed the maxim that a book should consist of examples. This is a book of examples, but it is necessary to clarify the sort of example these stories are. I have often used snippets of them in talks, lectures, and other writings, where they have served as *illustrative* examples, illuminating a teaching point about moral decisions or lending poignant power to an exhortation about the nature of suffering. But the "complete" stories, as I know them and now present them, have served a rather different role in my life and career, that of *paradigmatic* examples. The difference between the two types of examples, simply put, is that an illustrative example is an instance of something already known or formulated; a paradigmatic example, or "exemplar," reveals something new, previously unthought or uncomprehended.[5] That paradigmatic examples are revelatory reinforces Hawkins's claim about the potentially epiphanic nature of patient-physician intersections. These stories were or include episodes that were illuminating in just that sense for me.

Having said that, I must also acknowledge that what served as paradigm for me may be simply illustrative for the reader—just as, in fact, these stories are for me in the present, now that they are integral to my thinking. However, it is my hope to retell them with their original eye-opening power, while knowing that you may well see in them more, less, or other than I have seen. Your thinking with my stories may take you down paths whose entries I never glimpsed. You may find my actions, my lines, my interpretations banal, obscure, or plain wrong and prefer your own grasp of the matter at hand. It is one of the compelling strengths of narratives that they call forth different responses from different people; there is always more there than a single participant or observer can discern.

Of what are these tales paradigms? I realize, mostly in retrospect, that they have stayed at the forefront of my memory because they exemplified certain facets of doctoring that I had not previously grasped, either not at all or not usefully or not to the requisite depth. I am therefore making an epistemological claim for such encounters as I describe: these stories are representations of events and relationships through which I came to know essential aspects of good doctoring. Further, I would generalize that claim to say, more boldly, that this is the way good doctoring is learned or, perhaps better, is taken upon oneself.

The learning I speak of in regard to these stories happened not through discrete "lessons," even though it is tempting to use that term. Rather, the daily experiences of being in the presence of suffering and strength, of being called to meet vital needs, of being expected—trusted—to rise to that call, were transforming. Each encounter, each intersection of my life with one of the children and families I describe here formed my understanding of what doctoring has to be if it is to fulfill its claim of caring for the sick and therefore contributed to fashioning the person I had to become if I were to profess doctoring.

⋧ Attending

I FRAME THIS ongoing process of formation in terms of my learning to attend to my patients—learning, that is, to be an "attending." The attending is the physician primarily responsible for the care of the patient. The term sometimes refers to a physician in private practice but is more often applied in academic medical settings where it distinguishes the supervising faculty physician from the trainees—residents, interns, students—who bear real but lesser degrees of responsibility. Becoming the attending can be a fearful thing. She or he is always the go-to person for the resident confronted with a novel or troubling situation, the designated expert ultimately accountable for diagnoses made, treatments essayed, and prognoses offered. It is a weighty responsibility and a complex one.

The multiple, interrelated connotations of "attending" provide the structure for the stories to follow, which revealed those meanings to me long before I searched the dictionary for the definitions that encompass the many facets of the job. Like most of my colleagues, I came to my profession believing medical education to be the accumulation of knowledge and know-how and the attending to be the physician with the most. Thus, in order to become a good attending pediatrician, I would need to learn more—and more and more—about pediatric medicine, the diseases and disorders that afflict children, the details of normal and abnormal development, and so on. This idea was not incorrect; it was just significantly incomplete. It was only in becoming immersed in the day-to-day work of doctoring, coming to live at the intersections with real children and their families, that I began to recognize the limitations of an entirely knowledge-based construal of the task.[6] "Attending" meant a lot more than I had thought.

There are three meanings for the word *attend*: "to listen or pay attention to," "to wait upon (as a servant), be present at or accompany," and "to wait for or expect." The specific sense of attending as ministering to the sick is included within the second of these meanings in dictionary listings, but it is clear that each definition has its place in the spectrum of the physician's calling. In considering the content and order of these stories, assorting them roughly in chronological order, I found that my growing comprehension of the vocation of attending to patients seemed to expand from the first definition to embrace the second and then the third. Thus, the narratives in each of the three parts of this book are grouped under one of the core meanings of *attend* and of the act of "attending."

The reader may be struck by significant variations in length and dramatic intensity among these stories, at least those in part I and part II. Some are brief vignettes, others more protracted and detailed narratives. This variety not only recapitulates the actuality of diverse professional experiences but also displays a salient characteristic of revelation. Some epiphanies come as lightning strikes, like the Damascus road conversion of Paul; others play out over long stretches of time, like the years-long incremental transformation of Augustine.[7]

Moreover, some of the narratives are difficult to read, intense and troubling as they are in their sadness and sense of loss. Reliving them as I wrote was harder than I had expected. The children, their parents, all the conflicting emotions and complex burdens of each situation came flooding back as I let myself recall the details, the conversations, and the way it felt to be there, watching the truth of my chosen vocation unfold before me.

⪼ Part I: Listening

FROM JULY 1973 through June 1976, I was a resident in pediatrics at the Johns Hopkins Hospital in Baltimore, Maryland. The first stories come from those years of training. They cluster (loosely) around my learning to listen to patients and families, to hear what they are saying, whether verbally or otherwise, about their illnesses and their lives, about what they need from medicine. The learning curve is steep for interns and residents making the difficult shift from student to professional, taking on increasing levels of responsibility and, more often than not, grasping the nature of the responsibility only in the act of bearing it. On that sharp ascent, a resident may find, as I did, that certain patients reach out from their need and pain to grab their attention, to insist on being heard with a cry (literal or metaphorical) that pierces through the clamor of anxiety and weariness filling the trainee's head. Having caught that cry of need often enough—how many calls does it take before one's ears are tuned to the frequency of suffering?—a doctor will learn to listen for it, in all its shadings, even from the quietest, the least insistent patient.

Residency is largely regarded, with good reason, as the crucible within which physicians are formed, for good or for ill. It is a grueling period of intense and unrelenting demands—intellectual, emotional, spiritual, and physical. Now, in the first years of the twenty-first century, there is appropriate action afoot to alleviate some of the worst problems plaguing residencies, especially the traditional exhausting work schedule that diminishes the quality of both patient care and physician education—and, no matter what its supporters claim, neither mimics the sort of emergency responsiveness nor inculcates the level of commitment that is called for in many versions of medical practice. (Recent mandates reduce the resident's workweek from the 120 hours of my experience to a maximum of 80 hours, still well within the definition of *grueling*.) However, in the mid-1970s, serious reform was not yet in the air. With the exception of a few months in clinics and on electives, my three years of residency training were spent in an every-other-night call schedule, which meant that we all worked roughly thirty-six hours out of every forty-eight.

Against the unchanging background of demanding work and daunting realities of disease and human need, there is much that *has* changed in the thirty years since I was a resident. Medicine generally, pediatrics specifically, was much less technically sophisticated in the 1970s. You will hear in my stories from that time nothing about not-yet-imagined magnetic resonance imaging (M.R.I.) or even about computed tomography (C.T.) scans, which became available toward the end of my training and, as is true with many innovations, were used at first only infrequently and with misgivings. I shall speak of working in a neonatal intensive care unit (N.I.C.U.), but it bore little resemblance to a present-day N.I.C.U. The mid-1970s were early days in the field of neonatology; equipment was relatively primitive, knowledge sketchy.

We did have a pediatric intensive care unit (P.I.C.U.), but this level of intervention was also in its infancy. Many children who would now be cared for in a P.I.C.U. were taken care of on the regular pediatric floors of the hospital, tended by excellent pediatric nurses who were called on to care simultaneously for children hospitalized briefly for croup or tonsillectomy; children in for months—or even, in occasional cases, years—for treatment of chronic and life-threatening disorders; and children in the final stages of cancer, cystic fibrosis, or congenital heart disease.

Let me say now, for it may be muted in what is to come, that I learned as much or more about the care of children and their families from those nurses—and from the Child Life[8] workers who taught and played with the children, helping them still be children—as from my physician teachers and colleagues. Many of the nurses I worked with, then and later, took care of me as well as their patients, making my survival and growth as a doctor possible. I owe them more than I can repay, but I remember the debt each time I encourage medical students to pay close attention and sincere respect to these medical professionals who often know our mutual patients much better than we do, as well as each time I advise an undergraduate who wants to "take care of sick people" that such a calling may well be better realized in nursing than in doctoring.

The other significant difference in the residency experience between then and now is the level of responsibility given to residents. Thirty years ago, in many residency programs in the United States, residents had primary responsibility for patients, in and out of the hospital. The faculty attending physicians were nominally assigned the admitted patients but, though that perhaps entailed some moral liability, there was little sense of accountability in a practical, legal, or financial (necessary for billing) sense. Our attendings showed up a couple of times a week to teach us about the patients we chose to introduce to them. They were called "teaching attendings," apparently to emphasize that the position lacked any direct role in patient care. They did not make rounds with us; they seldom wrote notes in the patients' charts. They certainly did not oversee, control, or (except in the case of "specialty" patients with, for example, cancer or congenital heart disease) contribute regularly to the decisions we residents made about diagnosis and treatment.

I was fortunate to be in a training program that expected residents, not clinic staff doctors or attending faculty, to follow as outpatients the children with serious or chronic disease whom we had cared for in hospital. This practice gave us not only the opportunity to understand certain disease processes much better, by tracking them in their "managed" periods as well as in their acute exacerbations, but also—and at least as important for our education—the chance to accompany children and their families as they lived with their disorders, to observe all that "living with" meant and asked of them and of their doctor.

Soon after I completed my training, the atmosphere changed markedly, driven by demands of third-party payors that the physician services they paid for be provided by experienced faculty physicians and, more as an afterthought, by concerns about moral obligations to patients and pedagogical standards for students and residents. By the time I became an attending, the "teaching attending" with minimal clinical responsibility was a figure of the past. The attending physician now serves a role more like that of the senior or chief resident of old: close supervision, frequent documentation, and clear responsibility for all decisions. It is now most often a faculty attending, not a resident, who follows children with serious disorders through their outpatient visits, through the course of their disease and their adventures in living with it.

There is much, of course, that is very good about this change. When I look back on my residency, I am appalled by how terribly inexperienced we all were, how little we knew. We were a smart bunch; we all knew a lot about disease and its remedies. But we lacked the sort of deep and thorough comprehension that comes only with experience, and the most experienced physicians were seldom there to teach us what they knew. However, a major current challenge for medical education at the residency level is to figure out how to safeguard patients (and also protect students and residents from inexpert mentors and premature assumption of authority) by giving the most experienced physician the primary responsibility for patient care, while allowing trainees to gain familiarity with carrying the weight of accountability, to learn what can be learned only in practice and over time.

I cannot doubt that the experience of knowing these children, the ones I am now writing about, in and out of hospital, and of being the doctor to whom they and their parents turned was life-changing for me. They depended on me to know what to do, when to reexamine them, when to change their medications, when to admit them to the hospital and when not. They also trusted me to know about all sorts of other things, such as living with illness, growing up, parenting, dying, and surviving loss. It was their reliance on my integrity as well as on my knowledge and skill that compelled my entire and enduring attention.

≽ Part II: Accompanying

WHEN I COMPLETED my residency in 1976, I returned to the medical center where I had been a student, the Medical University of South Carolina (M.U.S.C.), in Charleston, to continue my training. After two years of fellowship, including one as chief resident, I joined the faculty. My primary jobs at first were as the attending physician for children two years old and older who were admitted to the hospital on the general pediatric service (as opposed to, for example, the cancer or heart disease services), and as director of the pediatric residency program.

In 1980, I became director of the pediatric intensive care unit. At the time, there were as yet few specially trained "intensivists" within pediatrics; I was called to run the unit primarily because I was the attending for most of the children admitted to it. I stayed in that position for seven years, until a specialist in pediatric critical care joined our faculty. For four years of that time, between the departure of our pediatric nephrologist in 1980 and the hiring of a new one in 1984, I had the additional task of overseeing the care of children with kidney diseases. My experiences during this time of caring for both critically and chronically ill children, among them the patients I write about in part II, built on and corroborated my encounters during residency and convinced me that attending to patients is a matter not only of listening but of being with them, of accompanying them—children and parents—through all the twists and turns along the paths of devastating illness and loss or transformed survival.

There are times when medicine has no more to offer a patient, no reasonable hope of restoration and recovery, of life without disease, or sometimes of life at all. Each physician develops his or her own mode of dealing with such situations—some ways more beneficial (for patient, family, and self) than others—based largely, I surmise, on the sorts of experiences, personal and professional, childhood and adult, that shape our individual approaches to the sorrows and impotencies inherent in the human condition. But if doctors are attentive and open to hearing the needs of patients and their families in that situation where "nothing more can be done," they must eventually recognize that there is never nothing to do. There is always the service of being present, of accompanying the patient and family through what remains—as guide, companion, assistant, or witness. This too is the work of attending, part of the ministry of service to the sick that is as much a definition of doctoring as is the knowledge, the technical dexterity, the professional demeanor, or the listening ear.

≿ Part III: Waiting

I LEFT M.U.S.C. in 1987 for the University of Virginia in order to pursue a doctorate in religious ethics, the step to which, I realize most clearly only now, I had been led by my patients. It was their revelation of the meaning of good doctoring that encouraged me to seek more effective ways of addressing their needs while fulfilling my now more firmly grasped vocation, by bringing new and different skills and perspectives to medical education and, more broadly, to understanding our moral obligations to each other.

When I say that it was my patients and their parents who set me off on this leg of my vocational journey, I speak truly but incompletely. It was also in large measure my students who showed me the way I was to go, by asking me to put my thoughts in order, to organize my experiences and responses into a teachable sort of wisdom. They challenged me to rise to their needs—just as my patients did—and, like my patients, trusted that my response to that challenge would be good for them.

During my graduate work and beyond, from 1987 until 2001, I continued to practice pediatrics as a primary care doctor in the university medical center's general pediatric clinic. The stories in part III come from that experience. As tales of primary care, they are in many ways sharply distinct from the earlier, hospital-based stories. They unfold over long stretches of time, revolve more around social issues than disease, and engage somewhat different aspects of my attention and abilities. I learned nothing so much from these patients as to wait. Attending became waiting from visit to visit to see if they would return, whether they took my advice and whether my suggestions helped, what new issues may have arisen, how the progression from toddler to schoolchild to adolescent was playing out within a patient's particular milieu, and how the children and their families altered, matured, fell together, and fell apart well outside my line of sight and influence. Often, I found, attending well to these patients meant being reliably present, welcoming, and consistent, awaiting their decisions to return for more conversation, advice, comfort, and help.

Listening, accompanying, waiting: these are the attending physician's basic tasks. Unlike the usual picture of the busy, knowledgeable doctor-in-motion, they suggest a quieter, more passive and reflective role. While this is certainly true, and I hope with these stories to suggest the importance of silence and space for contemplation of what each patient requires for her or his healing and relief, I also believe these tales say more. Attentive presence, compassionate attendance, and receptive attention are active modes of engagement that call for energy, devotion, and skill. All these facets of "attending" are essential in order that accurate medical knowledge, that other sine qua non of good doctoring, be used appropriately and well on behalf of those who come to medicine for succor.

PART I

Listening

Attend: I. To direct the ears, mind, energy to anything
—To turn one's ear to, listen to
—To turn the mind to, regard, consider

People don't have some Whozit's Disease, they have pain, they suffer, they lose weight, they throw up, they don't sleep, they cry, they die an endless death.

—Martin Winckler, *The Case of Doctor Sachs*

These are tales from my years as a resident in pediatrics; most are from my internship, the first year of residency. Internship is most physicians' first experience of intense involvement with patients, as well as of taking on real responsibility for their welfare. Suddenly, the facts learned in order to pass tests in medical school become the facts that may change (or end or save) a real person's life. The abrupt transition from needing to know in order to *be* right to needing to know in order to *do* right is unnerving and likely to be neither acknowledged nor guided. These stories find me struggling in the midst of that critical shift.

These early narratives have a rawness and unreflective immediacy that mirror who I was then, a novice emerging from the prolonged adolescence that higher education tends to enforce. I was relatively closed emotionally, trying still to be a good student/worker and not be overwhelmed by the physical and intellectual demands of the job, much less by its pathos. In some of the stories I seem oddly distant, a quasi-neutral reporter of the encounters, whereas in others I might well be described as overinvolved, a variability that may reflect my largely unconscious search for equilibrium in my relations with patients and their families.

In these encounters I am learning to pay attention to the truth of my patients' situations and needs as they know them to be. I am becoming someone who listens. I had to; the children and their parents were knocking, loudly and insistently, at the doors of both my brain and my heart. They woke me up. When I left Baltimore in 1976, I was not the same person who arrived in 1973. I had become a doctor: one who attends the sick.

Chapter 1

Telling Death

⚡ Joel

In July 1973, my first month as an intern, I was assigned to the floor that housed children two to twelve years old. One afternoon I admitted a two-year-old boy with serious congenital heart disease. Joel was quite small for his age, more the size of a nine-month-old, pale and listless. His cardiac abnormality was such that he would not live much longer unless some sort of palliative operation was possible; he was admitted to see if anything could be done.

After taking the history from his parents and examining him, I took him to the treatment room to draw blood for routine testing. The medical student held him gently while I did the venipuncture. Joel had been crying, with consistency if without much energy, since he entered the room; as the blood from his vein flashed into the tubing, he suddenly became quiet, to my relief. But something about the abruptness of the silence made me look up from my task—and I saw that he was quiet because he had stopped breathing. (Only later did I realize that the medical student, watching Joel's face while he held him, had not grasped what had happened.) We immediately began resuscitation and got others in to help. The more experienced senior residents took over from me, and I became their helper.

Joel initially responded to our interventions, but not for long. Despite our efforts, his weak heart could support him no longer. During the next few hours, while we tried repeatedly to get his heart to beat steadily on its own, the resident in charge assigned me to report to Joel's parents periodically. Two or three times I went out to the waiting room for the P.I.C.U., where we had moved him, to tell them that we were still working, using drugs, chest compressions, and defibrillation, trying to get his heart working again. When it became clear that there was no point in continuing the resuscitation, that the child could not be saved, and the residents were ready to "call the code," I was sent out to the parents once again to tell them so.

They were sitting together on the sofa, holding hands. I stood in front of them and said, "We're still working on him, but he isn't responding to what we're doing."

His mother looked up at me for a long five seconds and said, "Are you trying to tell me that my baby is dead?"

"Yes," I said. "I'm sorry." Then I left them and went back to Joel's bedside.

I did not know until she asked me that that was what I was trying to say. After all, my colleagues had used the same circumlocution: nothing's working. I had not yet translated that euphemism for myself; Joel's mother did it for me, and I knew she was right. I was horrified, then as now, that I had forced her to tell me that her child was dead.

⋩ Rashad

THE NEXT MONTH, I worked on the service with children less than two years of age, where another of my patients died. This little boy, Rashad, only eight months old, had developed a severe viral pneumonia of rapid onset. My senior resident and I spent much of the night he was admitted trying to stave off what seemed increasingly to be inevitable. Rashad hemorrhaged into multiple segments of his lungs, closing off those areas from effective respiratory exchange—a problem not fixable with the mechanical ventilation we were providing him. We labored to get his blood oxygen up to levels compatible with life, but all our efforts were to no avail. Rashad was near death with no reasonable hope of rescue. I went to tell his mother, who had recently returned to the waiting room after going home to see that her other child was being taken care of and to bring a friend back with her to continue the vigil.

It flashed through my mind, on the short walk to the waiting room, that I must not make the terrible mistake I had made the month before with Joel's parents. I needed to be forthright this time. This time, however, the child was not actually dead yet. We were quite sure he was going to be, and soon, but we had not yet stopped pretending that our actions might do some good. I could not honestly say "Rashad is dead," but I knew I needed somehow to make that impending outcome clear.

Thus determined not to repeat my error, I talked with his mother briefly about his lung disease and the implications of the hemorrhages, emphasizing the impossibility of overcoming the problem. And then, so aware that his death was inevitable and imminent, I asked if she would give permission for an autopsy. God forgive me. What could I have been thinking? I felt like clapping my hands over my mouth as soon as the words were out, but instead I sat there, at rigid attention, and watched her reaction. She took the papers from my hand and signed them, as if in a daze, and then fell from her chair to the floor, writhing and screaming, "My baby's dead. My baby's dead." Her friend reached out to comfort her. I muttered something unintelligible and inconsequential about his not actually being dead yet and fled.

I soon had to return because her baby was indeed dead. She was calm by then and looked at me without expression or comment when I told her Rashad was now dead. Leaning on her friend's arm, she walked back to his room and held him a while, kissing him and whispering into his ear. Then they left; neither she nor her friend had said a word to me since I had asked for the autopsy.

I had been taught nothing about giving bad news to patients or family members, had never seen it done before having to be the one to deliver the blow. (I think medical schools do a better job teaching about this subject now than they did in the early 1970s. Although it remains debatable whether anything can truly prepare a student for his or her first real experience of being the one to say the words, it must be a good thing to be helped to think about it beforehand.) I was not debriefed after either of these episodes, nor did I reflect on them seriously at the time. I mostly wanted to forget them and the humiliation

I felt at failing so abjectly at something so important. But, fortunately, they and my shame proved to be unforgettable—and crucial to my realization that the calling to heal, if that was indeed what I had taken up by becoming a medical doctor, was more demanding of my whole self than I had imagined.

Chapter 2

Pain and Longing

⇘ Milly

MILLY WAS A slim seventeen-year-old who wore her sandy hair pulled back from her pale, freckled face into a braid that followed her spine almost to the end. She had already been in the hospital a few weeks when I joined the adolescent service, in the third month of my internship, and took her on as my patient. Her first symptoms of back pain and trouble getting her legs to do what she told them had rapidly advanced to the point that she was now wheelchair-bound and burdened with the diagnosis of a large malignant tumor, wrapped around extensive portions of her spinal cord, inoperable. Radiation might provide some easing of her pain, some slowing of the cancer's growth, but there was nothing else to be done, no miracle foreseen. Milly would die within months, although I do not know if she had yet grasped that ineluctable prognosis—which is to indict not her ignorance but mine.

She was part of a relatively impoverished farming family in the western part of the state. This was to have been her final year of high school, but she admitted little regret at missing out on her schooling and less concern about whether she would be able to graduate with her class. I do not know whether this represented indifference to education or resignation in the face of her prognosis. Milly's parents and her eighteen-year-old fiancé visited part of one day each weekend. Other than that, she had no visitors, little mail, and few phone calls. Her world, perhaps never very spacious, had now been reduced to her hospital room and its television and the two wide corridors of the floor, which she circled over and over during the day, paddling her wheelchair, looking for company. Or, I should say, more often than not looking for me. She had a lot of pain. How could she not, with that crab chewing away at her spinal cord and most of its nerve tracts? I, the new young intern that I was, had followed the pattern set by the team who had cared for her the month before: a fixed dose of Demerol, given on a fixed dosing schedule. But Milly's pain did not seem to be governed by our schedules; it hid briefly after a dose, only to come roaring back long before the next one was due.

Her medication schedule was soon ineradicably imprinted on my brain, because every day, for two of the four hours mandated between doses of pain relief, Milly wheeled through the halls, calling my name. Her voice moved relentlessly through an ascending scale from whine to desperation, while never losing its distinctive slow drawl. "Dr. Mohrmann, can I have something for pain? Dr. Mohrmann, it hurts. Dr. Mohrmann, when is my next dose? Dr. Mohrmann, Dr. Mohrmann, Dr. Mohrmann . . ." I hated it; sometimes I even thought I hated her.

I was doing what I had been taught to do. The dose of Demerol was big enough; it was supposed to handle her pain. If it didn't, well, what could I do? I had consulted the pharmacologists and the books: yes, this was the right dose and the proper dosing schedule. Somehow, then, because the medicine was correct (i.e., I was right), the fault must lie with Milly. I did not exactly think through what that meant. Was she drug seeking? (Oh, yes, but not in the sense that label usually implies.) Addicted? Or simply insufficiently courageous, unwilling to just suck it up? After all, I come from a background—and a culture—that praises silent suffering and frowns on disclosure, much less complaint, of pain beyond bearing. And I had learned much more in medical school about doing things by the book than about recognizing and responding to a patient's actual distress.

I had to make myself go in to see her day after day, checking on her symptoms. She was always so welcoming, so glad to see me. Especially when her pain was under control, Milly was a warm, generous young woman, eager to talk about home and how much she missed everyone, beautifully dreamy when she spoke of her fiancé and their plans for marriage, curious about my life as a "lady doctor." She actually seemed to like me, and at those moments I liked her. But I dreaded the other moments, hours really, when, no matter what I was doing—dictating charts, talking on the phone, conferring with nurses—I would hear, rolling up behind me, the next round of "Dr. Mohrmann, fix me!" I was exhausted and angry, furious at having my shortcomings following me around every day and displayed to all observers, at being confronted repeatedly with my inability to do what I was supposed to do: make it all better.

After too many days of this, during our team's weekly care coordination meeting with the floor nursing staff, I brought up the problem of Milly's pursuing me for pain medication and admitted that I was distressed by it and at a loss to know what to do. I am quite sure I presented it as a problem with her behavior rather than with my doctoring. How can we get her to stop doing this so I can get on with . . . what? Being a doctor? Right. As though that were not precisely what she was calling me to do: be her doctor.

As soon as I raised the question, my senior resident launched into a long discourse in reply. I had seen little of this resident, my supervisor, since the month's rotation had started. He would show up for morning rounds, make some erudite assertions about each patient, criticize our work with predictable disdain, and disappear again for hours. Neither I nor my colleagues on the service wished to call him back with questions or requests for assistance, given his manifest impatience with our inadequacies. Now he proceeded to hold forth on the subject of pain control in his characteristic brusque and condescending manner.

Despite my bubbling resentment, what he was saying began to sink in. His point was this: For whatever reason, we—I believe he meant humankind generally, not just doctors—have the notion that people are supposed to be "stoic" about their pain. (Yep, that was me, all right.) We do not want to hear how bad it is, and we often believe and sometimes say, "It *can't* be that bad." Moreover, we—doctors this time—practice on the basis of odd and unscientific beliefs that pain relief can be administered on a predetermined schedule, that everyone's pain fits our dosing regimens, and that we, standing entirely outside the pain, can nevertheless "know" how much medication is needed how often, the "knowledge" that enables us to make ridiculous claims like "She's on enough pain medication; it can't still be hurting."

The aggrieved, still-a-student-working-for-a-grade portion of my brain was muttering bitterly, "Thanks so much. You've known for two weeks that Milly is on a fixed dosing schedule and never once said anything about it. You've watched her in pain, calling after me, and said not one word to me about how to approach the problem of relieving her pain." Had he done his job, I would have been spared the humiliation of this any-fool-should-know lecture delivered in front of the whole team, in front of the nurses whose respect I wanted more than just about anything. Yes, my primary response to his sermon focused on my shame and not on the fact that earlier intervention would have spared Milly so much suffering. In retrospect, I can recognize that an important part—perhaps the critical part—of maturing from the status of student into the profession of physician is making the shift from concern about one's own performance and reputation to concern about the patient's well-being. In retrospect, I can even acknowledge, with grudging gratitude, this resident's role in helping me to grow into my job. But at that point I was deeply angry and felt utterly betrayed by a system that I had thought was supposed to protect my patients and me from my rookie ignorance and inexperience.

The rest of my thinking, sidestepping the fumes of resentment and shushing the "Why didn't I think of this before?" inner critic, was focused on what the resident was teaching me. All at once I saw, with great clarity, that I could talk with Milly about her pain and its control. We could work out together what she seemed to need and keep checking with each other to see if it worked. And here was the best part: I felt certain that if I did have that talk with her, if she then knew I was going to be paying attention to whether her pain was being adequately suppressed, she would not feel the need to come looking for me, wailing my name up and down the halls. I could even tell her that I would check in with her at specific times during the day so she would know she would have my full attention then. Brilliant. Why did it have to be so hard for me to figure this out? More important, why did it have to be so hard on Milly? Is this what it means to "practice" medicine?

I had my conversation with Milly. She literally wept with gratitude and relief. I began to realize that the shame of not knowing certain medical facts was nothing compared to the shame of having failed her so unnecessarily. I increased the amount of Demerol she received, found out from her when she needed the next dose, and set the schedule accordingly. Then I checked back several times each day to see if that regimen was keeping the pain under control and adjusted the dose or the timing as needed. In fewer than twenty-four hours, Milly was a changed person. She was up in her wheelchair just as much, if not more, but now she wheeled herself into the playroom to watch the kids shooting pool or visited other kids on the floor or hung out with the nurses. And I loved to see her coming.

⚘ Crystal

AT THE SAME TIME that Milly was helping me become a doctor, I was taking care of another teenager on that service, an equally lanky young African American woman of sixteen named Crystal Meyers. Crystal had been admitted with newly diagnosed acute lymphocytic leukemia about a week before I came on the service. She was well into her initial course of chemotherapy when I met her and doing relatively well with it. An outgoing, irreverent teen, she seemed to be handling her hospitalization and treatment with an insouciant grace and an air of casual pleasure with the world as she found it. Even the inevitable medication-induced hair loss, which was already beginning to reduce her impressive Afro, became an opportunity for her to try out stylish and colorful head wraps. Almost everything that Crystal found at least minimally acceptable was greeted with a grin and a vigorous nod, plus the teenage catchword of the day in Baltimore: "Yop." Her gaggle of best friends, female and male, visited frequently, groups of them rushing in after school and staying until they had to be shooed out. Crystal smoothly incorporated them into her new domain, gathering other adolescent patients into this exuberant breeze from the outside world.

About halfway through the month, she began having headaches. They quickly progressed from occasional and short-lived aches to a constant, debilitating pain in her head that kept her in bed, face turned to the wall—a major change from the laughing queen of the ward she had been before. Her friends kept coming, but now they sat quietly with her, patting her hand, worry evident on their faces. At first we could not figure out the problem. Her neurologic examinations were all normal; her blood counts were no worse than we would expect from the chemotherapy, and she appeared to be rapidly heading into remission. We wondered aloud whether the pain was psychosomatic, the expression of fear and sorrow about her illness that she had been hiding behind her life-of-the-party façade.

Then, after a day or two of this, she developed a fever and a stiff neck to accompany the headache. The obvious next step was to look for meningitis, especially given the weakening of her immune defenses by the chemotherapy. There were indeed inflammatory cells in her spinal fluid, enough to make the diagnosis of meningitis certain, and the fluid also revealed the culprit: a fungus named *Cryptococcus*, one of the opportunistic organisms that selectively afflict persons with suppressed immune function. There was treatment available, but it was long and arduous, the results iffy and heavily dependent on recovery of her own immunologic integrity while keeping the leukemia at bay. The required medication, Amphotericin, had to be treated with care, the infusion bottle and tubing wrapped in foil to keep light from denaturing the drug. It usually caused fever and chills during the infusion and carried a significant risk of kidney damage. Moreover, Crystal would have to get this medicine three times a week for as long as it took to get rid of the fungus, at least months, along with the treatment regimen for her leukemia, which by now was virtually undetectable.

She did amazingly well with the Amphotericin. Her immediate ague-like reaction to it could be dampened, although not eliminated, with medicines given just before the infusion started. Her kidneys remained unfazed throughout the course of treatment, and the leukemia stayed away. Her headaches disappeared gradually during the first week or so of treatment. I was impressed, and so was she. Her stand-up comic personality returned, and by the end of my month on that service she was able to go home. We arranged for her to come to the outpatient clinic after school every Monday, Wednesday, and Friday for the two-hour infusion of Amphotericin, which I would oversee.

Each day that she came to the clinic for treatment Crystal regaled me with stories of her life at school and at home. She was quite a raconteur, full of life and thoroughly enjoying her adolescence. She giggled about the boys in tenth grade, almost all of whom were considerably shorter than she, and professed herself attracted to older men of eighteen or so. She would talk on, downing her preinfusion pills and scarcely noticing the needle sliding into the vein. The only clue that she was apprehensive about the procedure was the sidelong glance she gave the silvery bottle of "Amphoterrible." She knew that soon after the toxic medicine entered her circulation, she would begin to shiver and shake, unable to control the chattering of her teeth, regardless of the blankets we piled on at her request. It bothered her to no end that, because of the foil wrapping, she could not track the course of the infusion and thus, she imagined, steel herself against the coming rigors. After thirty minutes or so of this torment—during which she often tried to continue talking and even to joke about her misery—the chills would subside, and she would fall asleep for the rest of the course.

As she rubbed her eyes after her short nap, less garrulous now, long legs dangling from the edge of the table, Crystal would invariably ask through her yawns, "How much longer do I have to come here for this? Are we almost done? Didn't you say this would be the last one? Do I have to have another spinal tap?" Once a month, before her infusion, I would do a lumbar puncture to obtain spinal fluid to assay for the cryptococcal antigen. When the titer dropped below a certain negligible point, we would be able to declare the organism eradicated and the treatment ended. Finally, one afternoon after five months of her remarkably faithful compliance with such a difficult regimen, I could tell her that the last antigen assay was low enough to consider her cured of the infection. No more infusions, no more shaking chills, no more monthly spinal taps. Big tears sprang from her eyes. She jumped up and enveloped me in her long arms, then jumped back and started talking at a rapid clip about what she intended to do with her now liberated afternoons. She practically skipped out of the clinic, waving and grinning at the nurses, the patients in the waiting room, and every passerby.

After that, I saw her about every three months when she came to the oncology clinic for routine blood work and bone-marrow aspirations to monitor her remission. Sometimes Mrs. Meyers accompanied her, but most often it was just Crystal, hurrying over after school. As her leukemia stayed in abeyance and she felt quite well, Crystal the adolescent became increasingly resistant to the various constraints imposed by our protocol and by her mother. About a year into her course, she began talking of her longing to have a baby. A few of her friends had recently become pregnant, and she dreamt of having her own little infant to hold in her arms. She bought an infant shirt and some booties and brought them to show me. "Aren't they just so sweet, Dr. Mohrmann? I just really want to have a baby." She would look up at me through her long lashes, this tall, skinny, ebullient girl, and plead for my permission. Her mother, when she was there to hear her daughter's yearning, would roll her eyes and press her lips together, shaking her head.

Crystal's mother gave her daughter plenty of pointed messages about the foolhardiness of motherhood at the age of seventeen—only a junior in high school—and was adamant that she had no intention of taking a grandbaby to raise (a reasonable fear: when asked what she would do about the baby while she was in school, Crystal's answer was always "Ma can take care of it"). The tension between Crystal and her mother increased daily, it seemed, fueled by innumerable conflicts, only some of which had to do with fears or hopes of pregnancy. Once a month or so, one of them would call me at home, on an evening or weekend day when I was not on call, to complain about the other and to enlist me as an ally. "Can't you tell Ma to get off my back?" "Can't you make that girl stop acting so stupid?" No, I can't, I said in all the ways I could think to phrase it, while trying to smother my resentment of this invasion of my precious time off, trying to be a good listener and a professional explicator of the unfathomable ways of a teen and the inscrutable rationales of mothering, trying simultaneously to figure out if I was professionally obligated to play this role. More often than not, a few minutes into such a phone call, the other combatant would pick up a phone extension and enter the fray at full volume, making my contributions inaudible, as they perhaps deserved to be. Very unsatisfactory encounters for all of us, I expect.

Crystal definitely wanted *my* permission to have a baby, not only because she wanted me to trump her mother's objections but also because I had told her repeatedly that pregnancy was not an option for her at this point in her life because of her "maintenance" medication regimen. She was taking oral drugs to keep her leukemia from recurring, and at least one of them was an unquestionable teratogen, a toxin that would induce significant, even life-threatening abnormalities in a fetus. She simply could not have a baby, not now. At each visit, after I lowered this boom yet again, she would nod her reluctant agreement, head hanging low, big tears dripping onto her hands. And then she would spend the next half-hour adamantly refusing to cooperate with the procedures—especially the bone-marrow aspirations and spinal taps—scheduled for that visit.

Her resistance did not seem to be only or even primarily a tit-for-tat retaliation. Rather, Crystal was increasingly weary, and wary, of what we were doing, questioning the need to have such painful things done to her over and over when she felt perfectly fine—and besides, she claimed, there wasn't anything wrong with her anymore. Procedures that she had once accepted with little complaint were now accompanied by loud expressions of discomfort and copious tears. She would alternate between stubborn refusal and tearful begging, bargaining to skip the taps and punctures—all of them? one of them?—*this* time in exchange for taking them willingly *next* time. I was a rock. No change in the protocol, Crystal. This is essential for your well-being. The disease could come back anytime. We have to do this. A gentle rock—I held her hand, hugged her, sometimes even cried a little with her—but I always "won." She would ultimately give in and let me invade her yet again.

During my third and final year of residency, two years into Crystal's experience with leukemia and its trappings, the phone calls stopped. Crystal, now eighteen, and her mother had reached a truce of some sort, perhaps as Mrs. Meyers began to accept her daughter's move into chronological, if not psychological, adulthood. Crystal's complaints about the every-three-months monitoring procedures diminished, but so did her exuberant inclusion of me in her plans and dreams. She was as outgoing as ever, as apparently carefree and comical, but much less open. She no longer talked of her dreams of motherhood nor asked my permission for pregnancy.

September of that year was my vacation month. As I did with all my patients, I turned responsibility for Crystal's care over to one of my fellow residents for the month, explaining to her all the ins and outs of Crystal's course, including her wish for a baby, which I was quite sure had not disappeared, even if she was no longer talking about it with me. When I returned, there was a message waiting from the covering resident. Only a few days after I left, Crystal had come in to see her for an unscheduled visit. She was pregnant and scared because she remembered what I had said about the leukemia medicines' harming the baby. The resident consulted with oncologists and gynecologists and, on their advice, recommended to Crystal that she have an abortion. Crystal met this counsel with tears but no arguments; she had the pregnancy terminated within a week of revealing it.

I called Crystal. Mrs. Meyers answered and went on at length about her anger with Crystal for getting pregnant and her relief that it had been "taken care of" so efficiently. Then Crystal came to the phone. I told her how sorry I was that it had turned out that way and asked how she was doing. Her answer was only a flat and distant "Yop."

Over the rest of that year, I heard little from her between her scheduled appointments, which she continued to keep relatively faithfully. But twice during the year I was notified that she had been admitted to the women's hospital of the medical center, each time for pelvic inflammatory disease (a painful and dangerous complication of a sexually transmitted infection), for which she had sought treatment in the adult emergency room. When I visited her in the hospital, she was her usual outgoing, funny self—no longer talking about becoming pregnant, but using no birth control. She dismissed my recommendations in that regard as though they were beside the point.

When I left residency at the end of that academic year, her disease was still in remission. On our last visit together, we reminisced about all those afternoons of her meningitis treatment, how much she had come through. She looked at me with what seemed to be her newly wise eyes and said she guessed she had learned a lot since then. I told her that she would now be under the care of the resident who had seen her through her abortion; Crystal liked her and was pleased to know that she would be seeing someone she already knew after I left. We had a long hug and I wished her well, with more fervency than I could tell her outright. Four months later, the resident called me. Crystal's leukemia had relapsed. During the course of treatment, when her blood counts had dropped significantly, she contracted an infection and died quickly, apparently painlessly, with her mother at her side.

In the years to come, each time I cared for a seriously ill teenager or talked with an adolescent woman about her desire to be pregnant or worked with a young man whose chronic medical needs limited his yearning to be independent, I would remember Crystal. Her physical and psychological exuberance, her springtime urge to grow, was so evident and so evidently impeded by her illness, its treatment and prognosis. Hearing the depth of her longing and despair, feeling the fierceness of her fight for her vision of a normal young adult life, I learned to take seriously the incurable growing pains of teenagers who must also be patients.

Chapter 3

Variations on the
Theme of Competence

It was February 1974 and my second rotation in the nursery. These were early days in neonatal intensive care, and our N.I.C.U. was relatively rudimentary. We had no ventilators specially designed for premature infants. We rigged our own mechanisms for delivering positive end-expiratory pressure (a ventilatory technique to help premies keep their immature lungs from collapsing with each breath) by running corrugated tubing from the oxygen and compressed air outlets on the wall, past a pressure gauge and the baby's nose, to a bucket of water on the floor with a centimeter rule stuck in it. Also, we had no attending neonatologist to speak of, and no faculty physician oversaw the "normal nursery" for full-term infants, which was located in the women's hospital, two city blocks away within the interconnected multihospital complex that made up this enormous medical center. Everything in both nurseries was supervised by senior residents; the work was done by nurses and interns.

Each month in the nursery was a test of stamina, not only because of the every-other-night call schedule but also because of the hike (or run) down five flights of stairs in the children's hospital, over two blocks to the women's hospital, up five flights to the delivery room (the elevator was always impossibly slow in coming), and back again—a jaunt made a minimum of twice a day to see the newborns in the nursery, and usually many more times than that as we were called to attend deliveries or check on problems in the nursery. I remember clearly several instances of sitting in a rocking chair in the normal nursery at 6 A.M. after a night of work in the N.I.C.U.: I have just completed all the discharge physical examinations on the newborns heading home that day, and I am sitting to write out those exams and their discharge orders. I cannot stay awake to do this. Each chart shows the trailing lines left by my pen as I nod off in midsentence.

My colleagues and I would have defended vigorously our competence, our ability to rise to the occasion, to do our work well no matter what. Were we kidding ourselves? How competent were the physical exams I performed on those babies, how alert was I to possible abnormalities or signs of serious disease if, two minutes later, I could be incapable of fighting off the sleep waiting for me in that rocking chair? This, of course, restates a perennial question for residency programs in every field of medicine: how best to provide excellent patient care while ensuring sufficient education and experience for doctors in training, all in the face of the chronic problem of too few workers for too much work.

⅔ Sherry

ONE NIGHT that month the senior resident and I were called to the delivery of a premature infant. The baby's mother had a condition commonly labeled "incompetent cervix," an unfortunate name that seems to impute both defect and responsibility to the woman possessing such a cervix. She had already had a few miscarriages, fetuses lost in the first months of gestation because her cervix could not keep them bottled up in her uterus. Early in this pregnancy, she had had a surgical procedure to tie a virtual noose around the cervix to bolster its inadequate "competence." As a result, she had carried this fetus longer than any before, but now her cervix had yielded to pressure again and the baby was coming some six weeks before it should.

The baby was just being delivered when we arrived. It had a strong cry and looked vigorous but, as we examined the squalling infant under the warmer, we began to notice abnormalities. The child's head was unusually large, the sutures of the cranium spread wide, the anterior fontanelle ("soft spot") oddly compressible, like a partly filled water balloon.

Good heart rate, no murmurs, full breaths, good color. Only two vessels in the umbilical cord instead of the usual three, a variation sometimes associated with other anatomical abnormalities. Then we saw the baby's genitalia. The delivering obstetrician had declared the baby a girl, and so it seemed. But, on closer examination, "her" labia majora were large, dark, wrinkled, and incompletely separated: scrotumlike. The clitoris was enlarged, and we thought we could see the urethral meatus (the opening for urination) up on the underside of the clitoris, that is, more like male anatomy with the meatus at the tip of the phallus than female with the meatus farther back, away from the clitoris. Definitely ambiguous genitalia.

The baby's mother was still under the anesthetic—she had not been awake for the delivery—so we had a little time to figure what we would tell her about the gender of her child. We had been taught to say in such cases that the baby was "unfinished"—easy enough to believe in a premature infant, harder to buy when the baby is full term—a lay explanation of the pluripotentiality of embryonic tissue that can become either penis or clitoris, labia or scrotum, depending on the hormonal balance present in a particular fetus. The hormonal milieu itself is fundamentally dependent upon genetic influences, particularly the presence or absence of a Y chromosome. There was no way to tell in the delivery room if this baby was an incompletely masculinized male child or a virilized female child, not until we knew its chromosomal complement and, perhaps, something about its hormone levels. It is worth noting here that at that time—in pediatric medicine and generally—there was little, if any, idea that a dualist view, insisting that each human being must be either entirely male or entirely female, had been perhaps rather arbitrarily imposed on a spectrum of gender possibilities that are far more complex than we can yet fathom or allow. There were philosophical, moral, and psychological aspects to gender "assignment" that were never touched on in our discussions or in the relevant literature. Biology reigned, and we believed we understood biology.

And there was still the child's head to worry about. When we got the baby over to the N.I.C.U., we shone a high-intensity light beam from the back of the baby's head forward. The head lit up like a rosy lightbulb, the light shining out from the pupils of its eyes. This was not a case of hydrocephalus, in which the head is enlarged because of increased fluid within the ventricles (fluid-bearing sacs deep in the brain, which connect with the fluid column surrounding the spinal cord). This baby had *only* fluid where the brain should be, a condition named hydranencephaly. Unlike anencephalic infants—babies with almost no brain tissue whose heads are flattened, foreheads absent, with only rudimentary skull bones covering the bits of brainstem that may be present—hydranencephalic infants have fully developed skulls surrounding the fluid sac that marks the place where the brain should be, although they may have little more functional brain tissue than an anencephalic infant. The baby's muscular reflexes, steady heart rate, and normal respiratory effort were being driven, as they are in all newborns, by brainstem centers. But that automatic drive would not continue in the absence of higher brain centers. This baby could not survive more than a few months at most, and there was nothing we could do to give it a longer life. We called in the appropriate consultants to confirm what we surmised from that one simple test; they agreed.

The ambiguous genitalia were no longer a particularly important issue in relation to the baby's truncated future, but we still needed to have something to say to the mother. And to the admitting office. The child had been registered as female, based on the obstetrician's call. My senior resident called the admitting office and asked them to change the baby's plate—the plastic identification tag used to stamp all the necessary forms, orders, and such—from "Baby Girl Jones" to just "Baby Jones." But there was no policy that could possibly allow them to do that; everyone is male or female in this world. We simply had to choose one. If an error had been made, then, with the proper signatures on the proper forms, "Baby Girl" could certainly be changed to "Baby Boy," but that was the only available option. The indignant senior resident, failing to bully the admissions officer into changing her entire worldview, hung up, picked up the baby's plate and a pair of bandage scissors, and cut the word *Girl* from the plate, changing the child's identity at a stroke to "Baby _____ Jones." From then on, while I wrestled with the mother's needs and with daily decisions in the care of this slowly dying baby, the resident focused his energy on changing the long-standing hospital policy in order to allow the possibility of a child's being (temporarily, at least) neither male nor female. I do not believe he succeeded.

The morning after the baby's birth, I went over to speak to the mother, Ms. Jones. She had been told when she awakened that she had a little girl. I now had to tell her, well, maybe so, maybe not. Ms. Jones was a small African American woman, twenty-two years old, who had left school after the tenth grade. She lived on welfare, sometimes with family members, sometimes on her own, sometimes in shelters. She did not know, nor care to know, the father of this child, but she was quite sure she wanted this baby. She had wanted a baby for so long and had grieved the miscarriages. She had put a lot of hope in what had been done to keep her cervix closed and was now very excited that she had carried the baby long enough for it to be viable. She was certain that all would now be well.

I tried to explain the situation to her, fumbling through our mutual inexperience and incomprehension to find the words to say that we could not yet be sure if the baby was a girl or a boy. Her reply: "Either one is fine with me, but they told me she was a girl. I've got a girl's name all picked out, but I can change that if I have to. You just tell me when you know. When can I see her?"

Following what I had been taught, I tried also to talk with her about anticipating the difficulty of telling friends and family—the people whose first question is always "What did you have? Boy or girl?" But she brushed off my attempts: "I'll just tell 'em she's a girl, and if you change it, I'll tell 'em she's not a girl, she's a boy."

Then I tried to explain about the hydranencephaly. She did not believe me. She knew she was meant to have this baby—girl or boy—and that the child would go home with her when it was ready and do just fine. She did not need the baby to be smart; she assured me it would not need much brains to get on in her world. "When can I see her?" Any time, I said weakly.

Over the next six or seven weeks—the baby's lifespan—I remained the baby's doctor. I had two consecutive rotations in the nursery because I had traded my scheduled month on pediatric surgery to a fellow intern who was eager for another rotation on that service (I had done two of those in medical school, which felt like enough). Two months of nursery and N.I.C.U. work, all colored by this baby and its mother. I may as well begin calling the baby "her" now, because after a few days we decided—

gods that we were—that we would call her a girl, despite the fact that her chromosomes showed her to be genetically male. Our reasoning? Her mother had started out thinking of her as female. Then, when she saw the baby's genitalia, she was convinced both that she had a daughter and that we hadn't learned much in all our education if we couldn't tell that just by looking. Moreover, we knew the baby would die soon, and we had eliminated the possible diagnoses that would have required treatment of disordered physiology. The hole in her identification plate remained, but she became "she" to all of us (as, in fact, she had always been in our heads, if not on our lips), and we began calling her by the name her mother gave her, Sherry.

Sherry remained remarkably stable for three or four weeks, eating relatively well, moving around much as any other baby of her age. Her mother was sure that we were quite wrong and that, once Sherry was big enough, she would be coming home with her. The only sign that all was not right was that, despite her initially good appetite, she gained little if any weight. Slowly her muscle tone began to diminish; she made fewer spontaneous movements, and those she made decreased in range and vigor—and therefore she ate less and less. All through those weeks, her mother was there every day, all day. She sat holding Sherry much of the time, feeding her and talking to her, except when someone would interrupt in order to examine the baby or to let her warm up back inside her incubator. During those hiatuses, Ms. Jones would sit back in our conference room-cum-library. It was not the usual place for visiting parents to hang out, but we had made a reluctant exception for her after she had declared her adamant refusal to move to the distant waiting room.

I often went back to the conference room to write notes in my patients' charts or, when the work was light, to read up on neonatal problems and prepare for presentations on rounds. Ms. Jones and I ended up talking a lot. She remained impervious to our prognoses, so I soon gave up trying to convince her and just listened as she spoke of how important this baby was to her and how devastating the loss of the others had been. I came to know Ms. Jones as a tenacious but relatively resourceless woman—financially, educationally, and socially—who had cast her one hope in life on having a child she could care for and who, eventually, would care for her. During all the weeks of Sherry's short life, no one ever accompanied Ms. Jones in her daylong vigils in the N.I.C.U. or came to visit. She never spoke of family or friends. She came, through icy February and early March, with her orange knit cap, emblazoned with the emblem of the Baltimore Orioles, pulled down over her forehead, her thin jacket wrapped around her, her sockless feet in worn sneakers. The social worker's attempts to help her, materially or emotionally, met the same tight-lipped silence with which Ms. Jones faced intimations of Sherry's mortality.

Eventually, in our conversations, Ms. Jones began talking about her guilt, the burden of responsibility she bore for not being able to carry a fetus to term. Although she never delineated for me the faults that warranted such punishment, she was quite convinced that punishment it was, and deserved. She needed Sherry's survival as the sign of her forgiveness, the only sign that could assure her. I have no recollection of what I said to her, only that I tried to help her interpret events otherwise. With confidence in my scientific training, I was certain that "these things" had their explanations in embryonic templates gone awry, in cryptic alterations of genes in a zygote, in as yet unidentified forces that can lead the march of development down the wrong path. I had not yet learned that nothing in our science can answer the question "Why?" even as it answers "How?" and "What?" in increasingly complex detail and at levels approaching the atomic. I knew she was wrong to see Sherry's abnormalities and grim outlook as her fault and lost no opportunity to say so, in gentle and roundabout ways so as not to sound as though I were dismissing her concerns as nonsense—although I was. Over time, she seemed to begin to agree with me, to brighten up a bit as she became able to construe her "incompetent" cervix as just one of those things, unfortunate certainly, but not in need of absolution.

Sherry's condition deteriorated in her sixth or seventh week of life to the point that even Ms. Jones could no longer deny the changes, although she never stopped looking for ways to insist on an eventual return of health. Finally she tried one last avenue. She asked her sister to come and anoint the baby for healing. Ms. Jones explained that this was something her sister was quite good at and well known for in their community. Her sister—I had not even known before this point that she had one—arrived with two other women, introduced as fellow believers who would participate in the prayers that accompany the anointing. I asked if I could be present, and they readily agreed. The women sat in the conference room with Ms. Jones; I capped off Sherry's IV line (it had been necessary to give her intravenous fluids for some days now, as she had stopped taking formula altogether), wrapped her snugly in a blanket, and brought her to the conference room. At Ms. Jones's gesture, I laid Sherry in her aunt's arms. Her aunt unstoppered a small vial of oil, placed a drop on her thumb, and applied the oil to Sherry's forehead. She then pressed the heel of her hand on Sherry's forehead, her fingertips on her skull, and chanted a passionate prayer that Sherry be made well, that she live, and that she leave the hospital with her mother. The other women added their petitions and hummed concurrence with the ritual. Ms. Jones watched it all with avidity, repeating the amens, her eyes fixed on Sherry.

My eyes were also fixed on Sherry, because it seemed to me that her breathing had changed since I had taken her from her incubator. In fact, it now looked as though her breathing may have stopped. Just then, Ms. Jones's sister signaled the end of the ceremony with a satisfied look and a nod of her head that seemed to say that her work was done and done well. I reached over and took the baby from her, telling Ms. Jones and the group at large that I needed to take Sherry back into the N.I.C.U. to check her. When I placed her in her incubator, I unwrapped the blanket and put my stethoscope on her tiny, bony chest. Nothing. I watched her for a minute. No breaths, no movement. Sherry had died as her aunt anointed her.

The association of Sherry's death with the anointing ritual marks, in my memory, the beginning of my gradual journey into agnosticism about "coincidences" or, at least, about any facile dismissal of them as perceptual illusions or wishful thinking. In the years to come, I would observe so many instances in which events coincided in significant but inexplicable ways that I was compelled to set aside both skepticism and any claim to understanding. What I carry with me instead is a deep sense of wonder at the apparent power of the connections among us and, I suspect, between us and that which transcends humanity. I don't know what happened at the moment of her aunt's anointing and the women's prayers. I don't know whether or how those actions determined, in some fashion, the time of Sherry's death. I do know that my life in medicine was deepened and enriched by my increasing willingness to recognize the truly inexplicable and to leave it unexplained.

And now I had to talk with Sherry's mother, on whose face I had just seen hope rekindled by the prayers and invocations of healing. I told the nurses that Sherry was dead and that I was going back to tell her mother. They replied that Ms. Jones's sister and the other visiting women had left as soon as I took Sherry from them; Ms. Jones was again alone in the conference room. She looked up at me eagerly as I entered the room. "Those were good prayers, weren't they? I know they'll do Sherry a lot of good."

"I'm sorry, Ms. Jones. Sherry just died."

With that, Ms. Jones gave a yelp, sprang from her chair, overturning it, flung out her right fist, and hit me on my left jaw. I was taken off guard, but I was also almost a foot taller and much heftier than Ms. Jones. I immediately wrapped my arms around her to immobilize her and started saying soothing somethings. She collapsed against me and sobbed as the nurses rushed in, having heard the yell and the crash of the over-turned chair; one of them carried a syringe (of Thorazine, I later learned, a major tranquilizer). They stopped short when they saw us. I said, "It's all right. She's just upset. She'll be okay," and they backed out. Soon Ms. Jones asked to see Sherry. We went back into the N.I.C.U. Sherry lay where I had left her, but the nurses had cleared away her IV and monitors and had wrapped her back in her blanket. They pulled over the rocking chair so Ms. Jones could sit and hold her daughter. She held her for a few minutes, put her back in the incubator, and left the N.I.C.U. without a word.

The next day Ms. Jones returned to tell us the plans for the baby's funeral. I think she would have liked to spend the day with us, but could not figure a way to make it happen. So she made a little small talk, re-sponded briefly to our questions about her well-being, and left again, for the last time.

A few days later two of the nurses and I attended Sherry's funeral. The baby was in an open coffin at the front of the church; we watched adults drag their protesting children forward to see and even kiss the dead baby. Persons we had never seen in the N.I.C.U.—family members?—threw themselves over the coffin, sobbing. When Ms. Jones arrived, arrayed as usual in her orange knit cap and tattered jacket, she stepped up to the coffin and kissed Sherry, then took her place amid a crowd of women and men who reached out to pat her back, hand her tissues, hold her hand.

The preacher, a hunched old man with a quavery voice, took charge and led us through a few prayers. Then he launched into a long sermon. His primary message, repeated several times, was this: Whenever a baby dies, it is necessary for the family to examine what they have been doing, because such a death is always a punishment for the family's sins. The congregation said "Amen." I sank back in the pew, appalled at such a message, wanting to leap up and contradict him, knowing I could not. I could see now where Ms. Jones's certainty of her guilt came from and that nothing I had said was likely to shield her from her community's beliefs, their explanation for the bad things that happened to them.

≥ Daniel

DURING THE TIME when Sherry's life was dwindling to its close, I was called to the delivery room one afternoon on a semi-urgent basis. The little information I was given over the phone indicated that the obstetrics staff had thought the mother was having a spontaneous abortion—a miscarriage—of a fetus under the age and size of viability. However, the baby, once it appeared, was larger and more mature than they had expected and showed some vigor. A pediatrician was needed after all—but don't rush, they said. They did not expect the baby to survive, but the mother was anxious that everything be done, so they thought it would be politic to have a pediatrician pronounce the child officially "unsalvageable," as the term of art was, and probably still is, as though a human life were analogous to treasure hidden deep on the ocean floor, out of reach of human efforts to snag and retrieve it.

Silently, or maybe not so silently, cursing the bad judgment that had not involved us earlier—easy to do with the clarity of hindsight—I gestured to the medical student to join me, and we strolled the five flights down, two blocks over, five flights up to the delivery room. Along the way, I held forth to my captive student audience on the topic of interdepartmental politics surrounding decision making about fetuses on the cusp of viability.

When we arrived, a nurse pointed us the way to the room where we would find the baby. The room was dimly lit and cool. Over against the far wall, in a line of baby warmers—although this appeared to be a delivery room, it was obviously being used more for storage than for deliveries—stood the obstetrics resident, poking hesitantly with one finger at the chest of a very small baby boy. The warmer was not on; no oxygen was in use. "Oh, good," he said. "You're here. The mother really wants this baby, so I thought maybe we should do what we could."

Well, I thought, you *could* warm him up a bit; you *could* actually *do* something for him. I said, "Fine, here we are," and peered at the baby as I elbowed the obstetrician out of the way. He looked to be close to 1,000 grams and, at first glance, maybe at thirty-two weeks' gestation, which put him well within the limits of viability for premies in 1974. His hair was sparse and fuzzy, his light chocolate skin soft and dry, with some of the wrinkles associated with greater maturity, as opposed to the sleek otter look of the very young premie. Moreover, despite the resident's ineffective care, he was making spontaneous movements and looked like a live baby, not a dead fetus. I jumped into action that by now was rote. Turn on the warmer, check the baby's vital signs. No Apgar score had been given—they did not expect a real baby, after all—and it was now much too long after delivery (twenty minutes? thirty?) to think about that. Nevertheless, the clinical evidence used for Apgar scores was still relevant. Pulse, respiratory effort, muscle tone, color, responsiveness? He was making a weak, desultory effort to breathe, his pulse was slow but steady, and, although he was dusky in color, he did make significant voluntary movements. Not bad, given the circumstances. I placed the ventilating bag over his face and began forcing air into his lungs while I got some information from the resident.

The baby's thirty-five-year-old mother had been trying to get pregnant for many years. This much-desired pregnancy had been free of problems until she had been found on a routine examination to have an "incompetent" cervix and to be at imminent risk of losing the fetus. The obstetricians immediately made an attempt to tighten the cervix, but during the procedure she went into premature labor that could not be stopped. The baby was thought to be of a gestational age (somewhere around twenty-six weeks) and of a weight (estimated to be less than 600 grams) that would not be compatible with extrauterine life then. Therefore no one expected to need a pediatrician. When the baby popped out and cried spontaneously, the mother begged them to do whatever they could to save him: thus the resident's halfhearted attempts at resuscitation in the back room, thus the pro forma call to a pediatrician. It had taken the obstetrics team a while to decide to do any of that. Added to the time it took us to "not rush" over there, it had been more like forty-five minutes since the baby had taken his first breath. Having told me all he knew about the situation, the resident left to attend to the baby's mother.

As I forced oxygen into the baby's lungs, he began moving more, his color improved, and his heart rate climbed into the normal range. What was foremost in my mind, however, was the extended time during which the baby, so I assumed, had been without adequate oxygen. I looked up at the medical student, who was handling his own anxiety by continuous monitoring of the infant's heart rate with his stethoscope. He called out to me each minute the relatively unchanging numbers—160, 162, 158, 166—as though they were a litany of health or of success.

"What are we doing?" I wondered aloud. *Should* we be resuscitating this child? Even if he survived—and I was by no means sure he would— did he not run an enormous risk of being significantly damaged by that long hypoxic period? Were we just "creating," if anything, a baby likely to have severe cerebral palsy? But now the baby was breathing well on his own. What was done was done and could not be undone.

Had my automatic rescue reflexes, assiduously developed over the past couple of years, done something truly immoral here? I was entirely confused. This was not a subject that had ever been discussed in medical school or in my residency thus far. There had been the delivery I had attended the month before when a baby with severe hydrocephalus had been delivered vaginally instead of by Caesarean section. Apparently the diagnosis had been missed, disregarded, or downplayed—I do not know those details—and the enormity of the baby's head had not been recognized until it was inescapably apparent during the delivery. The extraction was difficult, to say the least, requiring a dangerous amount of time and effort to get that large head through the cervix and past the pelvic brim. The dreadful consequence of using the vaginal route was immediately obvious: the baby's huge head had been dramatically compressed, such that cerebral tissue had been squeezed out of the cranial vault, like toothpaste, through the gap at the bony suture lines. I could feel the skull bones, vertical like the sides of an open cereal box top, on either side of the baby's impossibly long narrow head, and then nothing but mushy brain for six inches above where the bones ended. The baby showed no signs of life and we decided not to attempt resuscitation. This was brain damage beyond speculation, this extrusion of cerebrum, squirted away from its anchorage in the all-important brainstem.

That case seemed clear; this one was not, and I had no senior person with me this time nor previous teaching in my head to guide me. I let the baby call the shots. He was breathing, circulating, moving: so be it. Let's take him to the N.I.C.U. On the walk back, the baby in my arms, wrapped in several blankets—there was at this time a certain casualness with premature infants that is well-nigh unbelievable today—I hashed over the problem in my head and came to the conclusion that, from this point on, we should just keep the baby comfortable and attempt to feed him. If he made it, fine; if not, not. But no "heroics": no ventilator, no workup or treatment for sepsis, overwhelming infection. It would be a blessing if some infection took him away quickly and relatively painlessly. We would have given him a chance, and he could either fight his way through or not. That sounded right to me, a good balance that honored the mother's wishes and the baby's theoretical potential but also took seriously the damage done by the long delay before adequate resuscitative measures had been employed. I shared my moral reasoning with the medical student who managed to look both suitably impressed and dubious and had little to say.

In medical school, we had been told repeatedly that soon we would be in situations in which what we did and did not know about, say, a resuscitation technique or the dose of a medication would determine whether someone lived or died. I was already beginning to realize that this was not quite true, that there were few pieces of medical knowledge or skill whose absence could make such a difference, especially given that residents generally do not practice in solitude. However, I was now also starting to see, with a sort of growing horror that I could not yet let myself examine, that I could, in fact, determine life or death through just the sort of uninformed and insufficiently analyzed moral decision that I was taking upon myself in this situation—a possibility that had never been broached in my education. I am not sure that the addition of instruction in bioethics to medical school curricula in the years since then has done much to alter that discrepancy. It is one thing to teach modes of analyzing and resolving identified bioethical dilemmas; it is quite another to form reflective physicians, able and willing to recognize and address with compassion, humility, and discretion the moral questions that arise continually in the day-to-day care of vulnerable persons.

The baby weighed 930 grams and was assessed to be of thirty-one weeks' gestation. He looked great for the next couple of days. He required no supplemental oxygen, made some attempts to suck a nipple, kept his temperature and heart rate stable and well within the normal range. His mother was overjoyed; she spent as long as she was allowed, sitting in a wheelchair beside her son's incubator, sometimes reaching out a finger for the baby—now named Daniel—to grasp. I was surprised but unmoved in my assessment and continued to be pessimistic in my conversations with his mother, trying not to let her get her hopes up either that Daniel would survive or, if he did, that he would be a normal baby.

On his third day of life, Daniel did not look so good. He was listless and showed some irregularities of temperature and pulse rate. In a premature newborn, this cluster of nonspecific signs is always reason to go looking for and treat on the presumption of sepsis. When the senior resident said as much, my immediate response was to call upon my earlier reasoning about the baby's likely prognosis to pronounce a sepsis workup and treatment ill-advised.

The resident looked at me quizzically. "How long a trial do you intend to give him? He's been fine for almost seventy-two hours. What else does he have to do to prove to you that he's worth treating? Have you looked at *him*, at Daniel, these past few days, or just at your own assumptions about him?"

I stared at him dumbly, and the images of the Daniel I had been examining, checking on, watching with his mother flitted through my mind. He looked and behaved like a real baby, an intact, albeit small and immature, baby. How could I have missed that? My supervisor's words triggered a sort of vision of Daniel's near future: of course, he could grow and mature and be able to go home with his mother. We would see if he had some problems in the future, but he did not appear to be severely damaged, nothing like what I had feared as I resuscitated him in that storage room. Right. Learn something every day. Thank God they don't let me make all the decisions around here.

I did the sepsis workup, which turned out to be negative, and treated him with antibiotics for forty-eight hours, during which time he returned to his previous vigorous state. His recovery of health was unlikely to have been due to the antibiotic treatment. Perhaps he had just been having a bad day, but with premies it may be impossible to know the difference between a bad day and impending doom. I began to talk with his mother about the future, to join in her joy at this unexpected gift of the child she had wanted for so long.

A few weeks later, after Daniel started gaining weight and becoming even more alert, he had another "bad day," another episode of listlessness and decreased appetite, this time accompanied by a slight rise in body temperature, that again signaled the possibility of sepsis—so another sepsis workup was in order. I explained the necessity to his mother and asked her to sit out at the nurses' station while I did the workup. She sat on one side of a tall desk, watching me work. Sitting on the other side of the desk was one of my fellow interns, who had worked in the nursery with me the month before and had returned to complete some paperwork. He and Daniel's mother could not see each other sitting there. He too watched me setting up to do the lumbar puncture and then made one of those collegial, joking remarks that we all used as part of our in-house language with each other. I do not even remember the terms he used now, only that they were disparaging to the patient and suggested that our valuable time and effort were wasted on the likes of him. I winced as he said it, shook my head at him, and said something that I intended to sound professional and serious, to signal to him that this was not the time for such banter. But too late.

Daniel's mother rose up majestically from her chair, peered down at him over the top of the desk, and said, slowly and forcefully, "That is my child you're talking about. What do you mean by saying that?"

The intern turned scarlet and apologized inarticulately, trying vainly to defend the indefensible, and then made a hasty exit from the N.I.C.U. Daniel's mother sat back down with a harrumph and a scowl. I apologized also, without attempting to defend what he had said or that he had said it. All that stuff we were so used to throwing around, all the jokes about our patients that we thought lightened our load but that, more likely, served only to make us feel temporarily impervious to the horror, the grief, the pathos of it all—all of it, indefensible. Once I heard it with her ears, Daniel's mother's ears, I knew, and I was ashamed. I cannot pretend I stopped participating in it from that day; I was much too interested in being part of the professional socialization going on in my residency to exclude myself from the argot. But I never lost the discomfort I learned that day, and I began monitoring myself—not only monitoring the surroundings for listening layfolk, but monitoring myself in order to avoid language that I would not be willing to use to a parent, whether there was a parent around or not.

There is much discussion now of a "dehumanization" characteristic of today's N.I.C.U.s, full of sophisticated technology that demands as much or more interest and attention than do the babies it is designed to aid. My experience in a pretechnology N.I.C.U., however, suggests that innovative machinery is not necessarily the prime culprit in obscuring the human status of these tiny patients. Dehumanization—blindness to or disregard of the humanity shared by patient, doctor, and family— begins, I believe, with the problem of being an intern: naïve, frightened, thrust into extraordinary situations with insufficient guidance or support, trying hard to be "professional" while having few clear models, the intern's supervisors having learned their professional demeanor in the same dysfunctional way. The pediatrician-in-training is then asked to care for, and about, infants whose prematurity limits significantly their ability to project a fully human identity, a personality. (Many nurses and doctors with long experience working with premies will insist that the babies have distinct personalities. I agree, but I suggest that the assignment of individuality requires a sort of optimistic projection on the part of the observer, a mature and humane decision to recognize a premature infant as fully human, regardless of the baby's ability to evoke that response.) It takes wisdom that many young doctors may not yet have acquired to see the human being in the premature infant, and another kind of wisdom to keep constantly in mind the incalculable value of these babies to their parents. The attainment of this kind of understanding is not inevitable; the defenses learned during one's residency can be a very effective impediment to becoming a wise, humanizing doctor.

Daniel got through that sepsis scare as well as he had the earlier one and had no other interruptions during the rest of his stay in the N.I.C.U. He gained weight steadily and eventually went home with his very happy mother. I followed him, as his primary care pediatrician, for the rest of my residency, another two years and a few months, and he continued to do well, without any signs of damage from those long minutes without adequate oxygen. He was a normal, happy, thriving toddler when I last saw him, developing just as he ought with motor and social skills entirely appropriate for his age. And it is still Daniel I think of when I am tempted to ignore the incorrigible limits to our prognostic skills, no matter how excellent, or to forget the remarkable resilience of even the smallest human beings.

Chapter 4

%———————%

Being Mickey's Doctor

NONE OF THE STORIES in this book is more wrenching than Mickey's. It was through my encounter with Mickey and her family that I most clearly and most unforgettably discovered the nature of doctoring. It is the grounding story of my career—perhaps of my adult life—and the one that encapsulates everything else I have to say. I remember Mickey more clearly than any other patient I have ever cared for, even now, some thirty years later. I owe more to her and her parents than I can tally. I have thought and rethought these scenes since they happened, but it took many years for me to grasp their fundamental significance in the understandings of doctoring that I bring to my work as a teacher of medicine, in the perspectives on suffering and human relationships that I bring to my teaching and scholarship in Christian ethics, and in my sense of myself as doctor, teacher, believer, friend, and family member.

I first met Mickey in May of my internship year. I had survived ten months: only two months left before reaching the relative calm of the second year, with its emphasis on general and specialty outpatient clinics, which I looked forward to as a virtual vacation. Coming back to the service with the two- to twelve-year-olds that month was something I welcomed. They were the age group I felt most comfortable working with. Procedures (placing intravenous lines, drawing blood, doing lumbar punctures) on babies and toddlers were more technically difficult, and the adolescents—well, they just asked too much and gave too little by my naïve calculation, plus that service had included a couple of patients who had left me exhausted and chastened. The fact that I had recently finished two consecutive months in the N.I.C.U. and nursery made this rotation look even better. I was ready for anything, fortunately.

Mickey had been admitted a week before, referred in by her pediatrician. She had had a particularly painful, refractory ear infection—unusual in a twelve-year-old—that led her doctor to check her blood counts and thereby discover the reason for her inability to rid herself of the infection: Mickey had leukemia. In the week during which she had been in the hospital, she had had all the necessary evaluations, had the ear infection successfully treated, and had been started on the standard chemotherapy for her type of cancer, acute myelogenous leukemia, or A.M.L. Of the two most common types of childhood leukemia, the other being acute lymphocytic leukemia (A.L.L.), A.M.L. was definitely the worse, less likely to respond to treatment, and, in 1974, offering a dismal chance of long-term survival. In the early 1970s we were just beginning to see that A.L.L. might in fact be a curable cancer, as it has proven to be. A.M.L. was notorious not only for the short lifespan of its victims but also for its association with dreadful complications before death, such as widespread and uncontrollable bleeding, and its requirement for particularly nasty chemotherapeutic agents—a terrible diagnosis, a grim outlook.

I do not remember our first meeting specifically, except that I was struck from the outset by Mickey's intelligence, wit, spark, and willingness to engage with me well beyond what I then expected of twelve-year-old girls. She was a tall, well-built child, with lots of curly auburn hair and a scattering of freckles over her nose and cheeks. Developmentally mature and athletic (she ran track at school), Mickey used to really enjoy food. Now, however, she was wracked by the side effects of the chemical bludgeons being used against her disease: nausea and vomiting, mouth sores, and a not surprising loss of appetite. She was not an uncomplaining child—no saint, but a real twelve-year-old—and made no bones about the fact that she hated this, all of it. She hated being in the hospital, missing school (as she was missed: her room was lined with get-well cards crafted by her classmates and teachers), and feeling sick all the time. More than anything, she often half-cried at me, she hated being talked about so much. Mickey had the shyness of a "big-boned" adolescent girl—I recognized that kind of deep-down introversion, having been one of those myself—and anything was better than being in the spotlight, especially because the spotlight in this case was more like a searchlight scouring the grounds of a prison compound.

The medical team made rounds first thing each morning and last thing each afternoon. The group included six residents and interns, plus a nurse (if one could get free from other duties to accompany us), and a student or two; in the afternoon we were joined, and led, by the chief resident. Twice a day a sizeable knot of people would stand beside Mickey's closed half-glass door, just outside the mostly glass walls of her room, where she could see us talking, watch me telling them about her, and register our unguarded (because generally oblivious) expressions of who knows what? Frustration and fear, indifference and weariness, love and concern? Who knows if I shook my head in despair of her future, there where she could watch me do it, or if she might have read my gestures that way at a time when I was actually despairing of my own future, having given a poor impression of my competence as the chief resident grilled me on the pathophysiological details of her disease and the pharmacological intricacies of its treatment.

It was only after a couple of weeks of this routine that Mickey mustered the courage, one day when she was perhaps feeling particularly body-sick and homesick, to blurt out, "I *hate* it when you all stand outside there and talk about me! What are you saying? Why can't you say it in here to me? I *hate* it!"

In my groping attempts to take care of her and of myself, and having yet formed no inner mechanism—of integrity? of confidence?—that would allow me to question or try to change the way things were done in this august place I had come to for training, I reached for some accommodation. I asked, "What if we did our talking down the hall where you can't see us? Would that be better?"

She muttered a grudging "Yeah, I guess."

From then on, when I remembered to do so, I had the team talk about Mickey while we were still standing in front of the room before hers. I have no idea, nor did I ask myself then, what the children and parents in *that* room thought when we began standing there so much longer than we had before, deep in earnest conversation—about them? Mickey could then watch us sail by, clipboards in hand, faces intent on the next task, no one acknowledging her with a glance or a wave. So determined were we to leave her in peace that we simply left her. She did not mention the issue again, at least not during that hospitalization. But I had reason, more than once, to recall the intensity of her anguished cry.

Two years later, I was once again on this service, this time as the senior resident, running those rounds that still went door-to-door, stopping outside each glass-walled room as though we were sightseers at the zoo. One day a woman accosted my fellow senior resident during rounds as we left our post outside the room she was in to move on to the next. I expect she picked him as the focus of her anger because he was male and probably looked as though he were in charge. She was a friend of the parents of the child in that room—perhaps a frequent visitor, perhaps on her only visit; I had not noticed her before and did not see her again. She was very angry, almost spitting, as she railed at my colleague for this rounding practice of ours. I do not remember her argument particularly, only the word she kept using over and over: *dehumanizing.*

After saying her piece, while my colleague looked at her sternly and repeated something about doing our job, she stalked off in tears. We glanced at each other, in her wake, employing that patronizing shrug and wry smile we had so easily assumed years before as the stance of the professional against the unenlightened. "Dehumanizing? What is she talking about? She doesn't have a clue what we're doing out here, does she? What's her problem?" My colleague looked as uncomfortable as I felt, but we never discussed it, then or later. In the back of my mind, though, I remembered Mickey and how she had felt about these rounds. There was something here to think about someday, when I had time and might not be called on to act in ways for which I lacked courage, wit, and energy.

During Mickey's hospitalization, I also came to know her family well. Her mother, Mary, was there most of the time. She was a native of the city, her speech redolent of the characteristic intonations and phrasings of her hometown (she usually called me "hon"), and a full-time stay-at-home mother. Her exuberant, enfolding personality was floored by this disastrous turn, but was no less embracing for all that. We hit it off; she took me in as friend and ally in this crisis situation, even to the point of letting me in on family jokes—both old ones and the new ones that present events gave rise to—and family idiosyncrasies. Through her eyes first, and then through my own, I got to know Mickey's father, Marshall. (Marshall was also called by his first name, Fred, at times, but the joke that seemed clearly to be associated with calling him "Fred" was never revealed to me. It appeared to be what Mary called him when she had a minor beef with him, and Mickey had adopted that usage, along with many other of her mother's mannerisms. "Fred" was always said with a sarcastic lilt and accompanied by a teasing needle.) Marshall was not around quite as much as Mary, given his full-time day job as a butcher at the A&P, but he came every evening, and, given my every-other-night call schedule, I got to see a lot of him. He was a gentle and affable man, in love with his family and the Baltimore Orioles, in that order, and over-whelmed by what was happening to his beloved Mick.

Then there were Flo and Joe, Mary's parents. Flo was a smaller, grayer Mary, equally intense and embracing. Joe, like Marshall, was quiet—and seemed older than his wife, not in such good health—with a down-to-earth manner and a sweet and warming smile. I saw Mickey's siblings only infrequently during this hospitalization, when they visited on occasional evenings and weekend days. Her brother Chris was fourteen or fifteen then, Joey ten, Jenny eight.

Mickey's leukemia went into remission just as it was intended to, a victory for the chemo, a great relief for all of us. She went home early in June, soon after I had left the service and turned her over to another intern for the rest of her stay. Before I signed off, however, I made it clear to the new intern that Mickey was mine and that I would be fol-lowing her through her outpatient visits, monitoring her disease. That is, as was the practice in this residency program, whatever rotation I was on, I would come to the cancer clinic to see her on her appointed day, and I would be the one to draw the blood, perform the lumbar puncture or bone marrow aspiration. I would also be the one to discuss with Mickey and her parents the results of those studies, plans for treatment, effects of medications, everything—the one they would call, at any time, if they had questions or concerns.

Moreover, neither Mickey nor her parents wished to have our oncol-ogist be their primary caregiver. Mary's initial encounter with the oncol-ogist had become the stuff of family legend, another family "joke," this one grounded in intense pain. On the day Mickey was first admitted to the hospital, Mary accompanied her. Marshall was at work and could not join them until he got off at the end of the day. That day was a nightmare for Mary. From the pediatrician's initial concern about the ear infection to the whirl of activity that followed Mickey's entrance into the hospital—lengthy history taking, meticulous physical examinations, blood drawing, lumbar puncture, bone marrow aspiration, even a tap of her infected middle ear—the significance of the day could scarcely be fathomed in the midst of it all, only experienced. The word *leukemia* had been uttered as justification for all the testing, accompanied by modifiers denoting uncertainty and the existence of other, less devastating, possible diagnoses. Mary had longed for Marshall's presence through this but knew he could not leave his job until later. By late afternoon she knew he would arrive soon, when they could face together whatever it was they had to face.

The oncologist—forever after in this family referred to only as "Les," a diminutive of his first name, which no one else ever used—appeared at Mickey's door, Mickey now asleep, exhausted by the unimaginable assaults on her body, the utter confusion of it all, the fever and the pain in her ear. Les asked Mary to come with him to the conference room to talk. She asked him to wait until Marshall arrived. Les looked at his watch and said he really needed to talk with her now. Reluctantly, she went with him to the conference room. Before he could begin, she said, "If you've got something to tell me, please wait until my husband gets here. Please don't tell me without him here."

Les started talking, reviewing the day's course, the tests that had been done. Mary interrupted him to plead, once again, "Please don't tell me anything before Marshall gets here. Please don't tell me this while I'm alone."

Les continued as though she had not spoken. He told her Mickey had leukemia. He explained the type of leukemia, the prognosis, and the treatment plans. And then he left Mary in the conference room, alone.

Mary told me this story late in May, when we were making plans for Mickey's discharge and I was explaining to her the follow-up routine. She was so relieved to hear that they would be seeing me on their return visits and not Les, who would be calling the shots from some distant control booth, so adamant that she did not want to see Les any more than necessary, that I had to ask why. She wept as she told me, reliving the awful pain of hearing that Mickey had leukemia and of being so terribly alone, treated so callously. "Why couldn't he just wait like I asked him to? I told him not to tell me, but he did anyway. Why?" I could only shake my head. What possible answer would suffice? I knew that, had I had the opportunity, I could have been guilty of a similar crime.

A day or so before Mickey was discharged, I came by to visit. Marshall walked out with me as I left and asked if I would tell Mickey her diagnosis—the name of her disease, as he put it—before she went home. Weeks before, I had talked with her parents about how they wanted to handle information, how much to say to Mickey, how much to dance around real issues. I had given them my naïve canned spiel about the problems of lying to children, who almost always know some version of the truth anyway and are deprived of the chance to talk about it if the adults around them will not acknowledge the truth. So now they were certain that they wanted Mickey to have the truth—how could they justify all the follow-up visits if all she had was the "anemia" they had been using as the code word for her illness?—and they wanted me to be the one to tell her. They would be there, of course, but they did not know how to say the words, so would I please do it?

"Of course," I said quickly. "I'll come visit this same time tomorrow, if you can be here then, and that's when I'll tell her." I walked off, quietly moved that they had asked me to do this, that they really regarded me as Mickey's doctor. Then I began thinking of what I might say, what it might be like to do it, and my heart sank. This would be a new experience for me.

Although during that year of internship I had had to tell parents that their child had died, those experiences could in no way assure me of my competence in giving bad news—quite the opposite. And I had never had to give parents a bad diagnosis, much less to tell a child of any age the news of his or her grim disease, to pronounce the doom that words like *cancer* and *leukemia* portended. How to do this? I spent that evening thinking about it, planning how to explain, at the level of an intelligent twelve-year-old, the nature of her disease. I worked it out in great detail. I went to Mickey's room the next day with a well-rehearsed account in mind, in which I would show her—even draw pictures (my pad was ready in my pocket)—how the renegade white blood cells pushed out the red cells and the tiny platelets and thus created problems of infection, anemia, and bleeding. I would explain something of how all the nasty medicines she had endured had done their work against her particular traitorous cells and why they had also made her so sick and made her hair fall out. I was rather proud of what I had put together, but that did not stop me from feeling apprehensive as I entered her room.

I had established a good relationship with Mickey, mostly by being around a lot, available and willing to talk with her about schoolwork or to compare the merits of her favorite nurses or to puzzle over the style of wig that would be both flattering and unremarkable. I had listened when she had something to complain about (which was, of course, often—we gave her plenty to complain about), and I had entered into her family's mode of humor and coping. Perhaps most important, I had been as honest as I could about what she could expect from a new medicine or test—or me. I wanted very much to keep her trust and respect, to continue to be honest with her but not to overwhelm her with information beyond her capacity to handle.

When I came into the room, I saw she was in good spirits. Now that she was done with the chemotherapy, she was feeling so much better. Plus, she knew she was going home the next day, and she was happy. The get-well cards had been taken down from the walls and packed away to take home. She was in her own pajamas instead of a hospital gown and wearing her new wig, the one her mother and grandmother had found for her that matched her own hair amazingly well, although it was styled in a way that was jarringly adult and formal next to her young adolescent face. She was sitting up in bed, talking with her parents. They all turned to me as I entered, and her parents' anxiety was almost palpable. It was clear there would be no small talk. I needed to get right to the point before Mickey started sensing the fear in the room.

I sat on the edge of her bed; she scooted over to make room for me. "Before you head home, Mick, we need to talk about when I'll be seeing you back for checkups. And we need to talk about why I need to see you back in the clinic. What have you been told you've been in the hospital for?"

She looked at me warily. "Some kind of anemia?"

"Well," I said, "you do have anemia, but the reason you're anemic is that you have leukemia." I was prepared to keep talking, but I saw her eyes widen in surprise, so instead I waited to hear her reaction.

She stared at me for a long moment, shifted her gaze to her parents then back to me. "But that means it can come back!" she wailed and settled into her now-familiar pout, the firm set of her jaw and protrusion of her full lower lip that signaled both her displeasure and the effort it took to be brave.

I regrouped, discarding my script. "Yes, it can. We don't know if it will; it may not. That's what we're hoping for, and that's why we'll keep checking you and giving you medicine at home—to keep that from happening, if we can."

Her lower lip trembled, then stiffened again. "I thought I was through with all this. I don't ever want to come back here again."

I felt that frisson of rejection that I was only beginning to get used to: the repeated, but still jarring recognition that, no matter how close I became to my patients and their families, no matter how intensely good the interaction, I nevertheless worked in a place that they wanted to put behind them forever—and thus leave me behind too. Now this child I loved, part of this family I loved, was saying the same thing: Let me out of here! How hard it is to keep their perspective separate from mine. My job is their torture. The place where I find such fulfillment and satisfying relationships is a place that they, no matter how sincerely they treasure the relationship, would much rather never have entered. The good of the encounter cannot outweigh, even though it may ameliorate, the evil of the situation. I keep forgetting that because, for me, it can and does. But that can be true only because the evil of the situation is not mine to bear.

I swallowed hard against my own feelings so I could agree with her entirely appropriate reaction and assure her again that her goal was, indeed, our common goal: to keep her healthy, out of the hospital, back in school, even able to run track again. I never got the chance to do my junior high pathophysiology lecture. The conversation was clearly over. I stayed around a bit longer to see if she had questions, but Mickey had nothing else to say or to ask. Her parents glanced my way, with shrugs and tentative smiles, as if to reassure me that I had done my best, and returned their focus to their daughter, as they prepared themselves to take care of her. I left, feeling both relieved that the deed had been done and troubled by how much I did not know about Mickey in particular and doctoring in general. Good grades in medical school do nothing to make one worthy to serve the suffering.

I saw Mickey, usually accompanied by her mother, off and on for checkups over the next few months. She gradually regained strength and started doing whatever twelve-year-old girls did during hot city summers in the 1970s. She continued to wear her wig, despite discomfort from the heat, as her hair slowly grew in. A few times that summer I was a guest in their house—lovely, embracing times of family meals, with lots of laughter. On one such occasion, Marshall brought home a batch of seasoned steamed crabs and spread them out on a table in the basement. Mickey's parents, siblings, and I tore into them, wielding mallets and picks with abandon, rapidly diminishing the pile of crabs. Then I noticed that Mickey was still picking at her first crab very slowly. I was concerned. I had thought her appetite had returned; she certainly seemed full of energy and did not appear to be losing weight. What was the problem?

Just then everyone else seemed to notice my noticing, and the teasing began. Apparently this was Mickey's traditional way of eating steamed crabs—excruciatingly slowly, carefully picking out every shred of crabmeat while avoiding every shard of shell and any taint of "mustard" (the oddly tasty name given to what amounts to the crab's steamed viscera, prized by some as a piquant bonus, like the condiment its name suggests, and disdained by others who cannot forget its previous role in the crab's life). They were quite used to Mickey's eating a single crab in the time it took the rest of us to down four or five. She smiled slightly at their scoffing, holding herself above it, focused on the fine art of crustacean demolition. It was good to see her being recognizably, irreducibly Mickey among those who knew and loved her, idiosyncrasies and all. It was a very happy evening.

Late in October came the clinic visit I had dreaded. Mickey felt fine and was well into the school year, rejoicing in normalcy regained. It was a routine checkup, but this time the lab results showed that the leukemia had returned: the remission was over. Les was there, and we told Mickey and Mary together that she would have to come back into the hospital for another round of intensive chemotherapy. Mickey was stunned. She and her mother shed a few tears but then went about the business of facing the next step, starting the climb all over again. In retrospect, I suspect they were resigned to having to go through it all again, but expected the same outcome as before. Neither of them could have known what I knew: the first remission was the only remission. In 1974, for a patient's A.M.L. to relapse was to lose virtually all hope of cure or even long-term remission. Mickey's first remission—the first was almost always the longest—had lasted fewer than five months. The most we could hope for now was a few more good months at home, nothing more. I did not say that to them, and I believe they were not thinking it. I began then to comprehend that knowledge itself is one of the burdens a doctor is obligated to bear.

As it happened, that month I was once again working on the floor to which Mickey would be readmitted. She would be my inpatient again. When she arrived in the ward a few hours later, after she and Mary went home long enough to pack a bag and notify the rest of the family, I took her into the treatment room to do her admission physical examination and get started on the tests and treatments that were dictated by the study protocols for her disease. This time the chemotherapy would be more brutal than before, but I did not intend to warn her of that. She would find out for herself in time; no need to have to suffer through the anticipation of it too.

While I did the exam in the treatment room, Mary sat in the hospital room that would be Mickey's, talking to the senior resident, giving Mickey's history yet again. Mickey and I chatted some as I worked, but it was awkward—I resolutely cheery, Mickey uncertain, quiet, a bit disoriented. In a weak attempt to take some of the bite out of this hospitalization, I talked of nurses and Child Life workers she would enjoy seeing again. I suspect that ploy triggered her question: "What about LaTanya? How's she doing?"

Eight-year-old LaTanya, who had also had leukemia, had been Mickey's roommate for a few weeks in May, until each girl had required a room of her own to protect her from infection. Mickey and her mother had "adopted" LaTanya, whose own mother could not be with her during weekdays, and the two girls chatted, played board games, watched TV, complained about the food, and cried over needle sticks together.

LaTanya's disease had not gone into remission. She had never left the hospital, but had died during the summer.

"She died, Mickey. I'm sorry. It happened a couple of months ago."

"She died!" Mickey's eyes practically jumped out of her head as she stared at me in stricken disbelief. "Am I going to die?"

Oh, no. Not that question. I'm not ready for this. She's boring holes through me with her eyes. There is no evasion possible. I cannot deflect this. Oh God, I want to. I'm the one she's asking. I'm the one who has to answer. Any number of possible replies zipped through my head, each discarded as soon as it appeared: too dishonest, too hokey, too obviously an escape. This girl deserves better from me. Do I have better to give her?

"You have a disease people can die from, Mick, but that's not what's happening right now. And we're doing everything we can to be sure that doesn't happen. LaTanya did have leukemia, but it was a different kind from yours, and she didn't respond to the treatment. The medicines didn't work for her. They've been working for you, and we think they'll work again."

"Okay. They'd better work," she said with all the defiance of a child who knows she is trapped in an unfair world.

She never asked me The Question again. Over the next few weeks, she talked around the subject with an art therapist who helped her draw and paint her way out of the isolation that had to be imposed to protect her from infection as her immune defenses succumbed to the chemotherapy. She even, so the therapist reported, got to the point of calling it "The Big Question," acknowledging its existence in the room and in her mind, but she did not ask directly again about the possibility of her dying—not until a week or so before death came, and then it was to her parents that she posed it.

Mickey was readmitted to the hospital, and the routine began again. Toxic medicines, intravenous lines that were increasingly difficult to place and maintain, nausea and vomiting, days of feeling rotten—better just slept away—alternating with days of feeling feisty and homesick at the same time. The room filled quickly with cards from classmates again, taped to every available space on walls and curtains alike. Within a week of her admittance, her white blood cell counts were too low to risk exposing her to all the germs abroad on our lips and our hands, which meant protective isolation. Everyone who entered her room, family and staff alike, donned yellow gowns and surgical face masks covering nose and mouth. She did not like it a bit, but soon gave up complaining; it took too much energy, and she never won.

On Halloween night I was on call, my last night on before leaving the service for an elective month without call, a precious rarity in this residency. Flo, Mickey's grandmother, came to be with her while Mary and Marshall stayed home so the younger children could go trick-or-treating. Flo had decided that Halloween needed to come to Mickey too—so she brought *me* a costume. Black curly wig, black lacy shawl, elbow-length black gloves: I was to be a "lady of the evening" that night, she informed me. Mickey was delighted; she seemed to think it the perfect role for me. I looked askance at Flo's bagful of black clothing, especially at the rather dreadful wig, but neither Flo nor Mickey would let me back out. I still have the photo Flo took of me in Mickey's room, in yellow gown and surgical mask, long black gloves, absurd black wig, the black shawl draped suggestively over my shoulders. I am standing against a backdrop of some of the numerous get-well cards plastering the room. My left hand is resting coyly on a carved pumpkin. Perched on top of the black wig is my addition to the costume, one of my prized possessions: a dime-store nurse's cap emblazoned with "Dr. Mohrmann, R.N."—a gift the N.I.C.U. nurses had given me that spring at the end of my two-month stint there.

The three of us laughed—or, more accurately, I pranced and postured, Flo made bawdy remarks, and Mickey guffawed—until I was called away to the telephone. When I left the room still in full regalia, we laughed even harder. I came back later to tell them about the odd looks I had received from the other patients and their parents as I traipsed through the halls. No one could figure out who that odd woman was.

With Mickey's reentry into the hospital, her siblings began to fall apart in their own ways. Chris, her older brother, had been given the opportunity to attend an excellent prep school just outside the city. He boarded there during the week and came home on weekends. But, as he later said quite clearly, he could not tolerate being away from home while Mickey was so sick, so he ran away from school one night and turned up at home, refusing to go back. Joey began doing poorly, academically and behaviorally, in his school, a real change for him. Jenny went skating and broke her leg.

I asked Mary, after she recited this litany of mishaps to me, what the children knew about Mickey's illness. She said that she and Marshall had told Chris Mickey's diagnosis and thought he probably understood what was going on, although he did not talk about it. They had not told the younger ones anything except that Mickey was sick; they were not sure what they knew or guessed. Later I talked with Kathryn, the social worker on the oncology service, who made the wise suggestion that she and I offer a home visit to talk with the children. Mary and Marshall jumped at the suggestion, pleased and relieved that we would take on the task they had been avoiding, while knowing it had to be done. We set a date for one evening early the following week.

When we arrived at their house, Mary ushered us into the dining room, and we all sat around the table, with coffee and sodas and cake before us, to have our conversation. Kathryn and I had done some earlier planning so, on cue, I launched into an explanation of Mickey's illness, including an abbreviated version of the pathophysiology lecture I had prepared for her in June but had never delivered. I explained the treatment, why she had to be in the hospital so long, and what the isolation was intended to accomplish. And then I told them the possible outcomes, including death, while trying to be as optimistic as I could. They listened attentively; no one fidgeted or giggled. Kathryn spoke directly to Chris about how difficult it must have been for him to be away from home when so much was going on. She acknowledged the significant additional pain for the children caused by their parents' being so preoccupied with Mickey's illness and by the loss of the usual routines and expectations of life at home.

Joey, who was sitting next to me, had kept his head down throughout the discussion; he had not touched the cake on his plate. I looked at him and, all at once, knew what else needed saying. To the table in general I said, "You know, a lot of times kids say mean things to each other. Things like, 'I wish you were dead.' Or sometimes you just think it and don't say it. I want you guys to know that saying or thinking that kind of stuff doesn't make people sick. Mickey did not get sick because you wished something bad on her. This isn't your fault."

Joey expelled a great rush of air and slid halfway down in his chair like a man who had just been acquitted by the jury. I cannot pretend that everything was rosy for the children from that night on—of course it was not—but Joey's school performance improved noticeably, and there was no further trouble among Mickey's siblings.

Mickey was another matter. I had told her ahead of time about the planned meeting at her house, why we thought it was a good idea, and what I was going to tell her brothers and sister about her illness. She had little to say, just nodded solemnly as she received the information. The day after the meeting she was tearful and angry. "I don't see why you had to go talk to them. What did you tell them about me? Why aren't you telling me those things?"

"I didn't tell them anything I haven't told you, Mick." (That was not quite true; I had not been nearly as forthright with her about the possibility of death.) I went over most of what I had talked about the night before, but she was not mollified.

"But why did you do it? I hate being talked about." And so it dawned on me. This was like the problem with making rounds outside her room, talking about her instead of to or with her, treating her as patient on display and not as Mickey, the human being most intimately involved in the subject matter of the discussion. But there was more. Her separation from her family (she saw her siblings no more than twice a week during this time) was a significant part of her suffering, and I had intensified it by going to her house—something she could not do—and talking with them *about* her, as though she were no longer part of the family. Worse, I had talked mostly about her *disease*, as though it had now taken the place of their sister Mickey. I could only apologize and assure her, although I doubt she was reassured, that I was not hiding anything from her, not sharing information with Chris and Joey and Jenny that I was not also giving her.

Soon after that the treatment and the disease together began to take their toll. I left the service at the beginning of November to begin a "reading" elective I had arranged months before with our neonatologist. It was to be an opportunity to immerse myself in what was known about the health problems and medical care of premature infants. I did end up reading a couple of books and many journal articles about premies that month, but my more enduring educational experience took place in the P.I.C.U., where Mickey took up residence early in November.

Mickey's move to the P.I.C.U. was deemed necessary because of the many devastating consequences of leukemia and its fearful treatment, which could include infection, bleeding, neurologic abnormalities . . . the list goes on. At some point she became much less alert than she had been, and it was concluded that she had bled someplace, probably several places, in her brain. The severity of her illness and the combination of fears and distresses, ours and hers, resulted in her transfer from the room with all the bits of home in it to the room with nothing but cold tiled walls and a television—card art, stuffed animals, and flowers not allowed.

One night soon after her transfer I was in the P.I.C.U. with her. I cannot now recall if I was taking call for someone else, or just there because I wanted to be. It was late, 1 or 2 A.M.; her parents had gone home hours before. Something about Mickey that night made me think her death was imminent. In retrospect, I wonder if what I realized that night was that her death was inevitable. Perhaps I had not let myself think that far before. Whatever the illumination was, I remembered the importance to Mickey and her family of their Roman Catholic faith—the children enrolled in parochial school, the family an integral part of the parish, the priests spoken of familiarly as vital parts of their lives. (Among those priests was the one whom Mickey insisted looked like Ted Baxter, a character on the then-popular *Mary Tyler Moore Show.* If I was around when he came to visit, I inevitably got an elbow nudge and wink from whichever family member was standing closest to me and was invited to participate in the general, gentle laughter after he left. He did look like Ted Baxter, complete with the air of unwarranted self-confidence that characterized that bumbling, pompous TV newscaster. Mick was right on target.)

That night, watching a stuporous Mickey take big, halting breaths, I feared she was dying and, all of a sudden, I was certain that it was necessary to call a priest—now. My reasoning, such as it was, was that it would be important to Mary and Marshall to know that she had had last rites: thus my knowledge of Catholicism. But I did not know the names of the priests ("Ted Baxter" would surely not do) nor even the name of the parish. So, mea maxima culpa, I called Mickey's parents, in the dead of night, to ask the name of their priest.

"No, she hasn't changed any. No, nothing's happened. No, you don't need to come. I just thought that, as sick as she is, anything could happen any time, and I thought it would be important for her and for you to have had the priest here."

"Are you talking about last rites?!"

"I guess so, although I don't really think you need to worry."

They gave me the priest's name. I called him and he came right over. What could I have been thinking? Who knows? How does one learn, in this business, not to mistake one's own epiphanies for meaningful changes in the lives of patients? I expect this was some mix of wanting to do it all correctly, to be the complete doctor, sensitive to this family's particular needs, not missing an opportunity to care for them, coupled with my unacknowledged, indeed unrecognized, difficulty dealing with the midnight realization that Mickey was going to die sooner rather than later.

I told the priest my concerns, as far as I understood them at that moment, and he explained to me, quite patiently given the hour, that the issue was not "last rites," as popularly understood by non-Catholics such as I, but prayers for the sick—which were always appropriate and carried no necessary association, subtle or otherwise, with imminent death. That sounded just right to me, as I had now begun to think I might have erred in calling him out in the middle of the night. He went into her room to pray.

Just then Mickey's parents came rushing in from the elevators. "What's going on? Is the priest here? What's happening with Mickey?"

"He's in there now. She's the same as when you left this evening. You can go in with him if you want."

Marshall went in to join the priest in his prayers. Mary just shook her head silently and retreated to the waiting room—to wait. I sat there with her, but there was little to say. I had no way to explain, much less justify, what I had done to them that night. I was still not sure that it had been an entirely wrong thing to do, but it had certainly mushroomed out of my control, gone well beyond what I had imagined when I embarked upon this putatively sensitive acknowledgment of what I presumed to be their religious concerns. What an ass! In that episode I recognize the seeds of my later insistence upon clarity on such matters long before they were called for. It would take more clumsy errors—perhaps none of this magnitude, but errors nonetheless—before that lesson would alter my behavior and my understanding, but I have never forgotten this scene or the feeling of having intensified their suffering because of my needs, my ignorance, and my ineptness.

The priest—he was not Ted Baxter but one of the younger clergy, the one Mickey thought was drop-dead gorgeous—came to find Mary after he had finished the prayers. He squatted in front of Mary and put his hand on hers. She had been crying, not something she did much of when others were around, and she looked up at him with as bleak a face as I had seen on a human being. With great conviction, she said softly, "I hate this place."

Immediately, the young priest said, "No, you don't, Mary. This is a good place."

"I do. I do. I hate it."

To my surprise, I found myself saying, "Of course she does. Of course you do, Mary. How could you not?"

The priest flicked a glance at me, rose to his feet, patted Mary's hand one last time, and left. And at that moment I hated the place too, and me in it.

Mickey lived another two weeks or so after that night. The days that remained were a gray, unchanging scene. We had stopped Mickey's chemotherapy because her counts were so low—and because we were, in essence, waiting for her to die from the neurologic damage wrought by the bleeding, if not from some new assault. There was no longer any reasonable hope that she would survive for long, much less that she would be able to return to anything like her old self. Not that we ever said as much, to each other or to her parents. We just settled into the grim routine of daily neurologic exams and blood counts (why? because that was the routine), donning our yellow gowns and surgical masks each time we entered her P.I.C.U. room.

Mickey slept a lot or, perhaps more accurately, slipped in and out of consciousness. When she was awake, she was coherent, mostly; she knew people and could still muster a smile at a Ted Baxter joke. At some point she let us know that she could no longer see anything except some contrast of light and darkness. She did not announce this as a sudden or frightening revelation, just a point made in passing, thinking we might be interested. Again, bleeding was the culprit; her retinas could not be seen for the blood that filled her eyeballs. As the consulting ophthalmologist said rather bluntly, it did not really matter whether the bleeding was only in her eyes or also in the part of her brain that received nerve impulses from the eyes and presented them to the rest of the brain as visual images. She was dying; nothing was going to be done, or could be done, about her vision. She was in no apparent pain, for which I remain deeply grateful, especially given how little we understood about pain control in 1974. Mickey spent the last two weeks of her life quite blind and mostly asleep.

Each day I joined Mary for a while as she kept vigil by Mickey's bedside, each of us wearing the regulation isolation gown and face mask, talking little. On one of those days, Mickey woke up while I was there, and we talked a bit, mostly my checking to see if she was comfortable, if she needed anything. I stood by the bed, my hand resting lightly on her pale, bald scalp. She mumbled, "I want to kiss someone."

I thought I had not heard her correctly. "What did you say, Mick?"

Clearly and forcefully this time, with a tinge of desperate tears in it: "I want to kiss someone." I felt my heart break. So this is what it feels like, I thought.

I called Mary over and told her to take her mask off, that her daughter wanted a kiss.

"Is it all right?"

"You bet it is. Go right ahead."

Mary untied the mask and let it drop. She bent down and kissed her daughter's swollen, crusted lips and then put her cheek on Mickey's for a long moment. Mickey smiled and slipped back into sleep. Mary turned away from me as she redid her mask. Watching her, I received another revelation of the obvious.

"Mary," I said, "you don't need to put it back on. You've kissed her. What's the point?"

Indeed, what was the point? We knew she was dying. We knew that infection could be the final blow, as much as bleeding could be, but that the name of the final blow did not much matter. Why maintain this isolation, keeping her from the human contact she needed? Why had her last sight of her parents been of their eyes only, the rest of their faces hidden, their old familiar clothes covered, their hands hesitant to hold hers lest they harm her somehow? Why indeed? I began, tentatively at first, then with increasing conviction, to lobby with the residents on the service to end the isolation. Yes, it was what one did for someone with counts as low as hers, but to what end in this case? How could it be justified? They were skeptical, and I too was a bit afraid of this novel idea. Although her doctors resisted overturning established protocol, I encouraged Mary and Marshall not exactly to flout the rules, but not to hold back from holding, touching, and kissing their child.

Kathryn, the social worker with whom I had made the visit to Mickey's home, also kept vigil with Mary during those days. As her schedule allowed, she would join Mary at Mickey's bedside for an hour or so. Sometimes I was there too and observed the behavior that Mary talked about later. Kathryn and Mary would sit quietly, saying little. This was not a venue for chatting; it was a sacred space of watching and waiting. Periodically, Kathryn would sigh, shake her head back and forth a few times, and murmur into the full silence, "I don't know." She would then be quiet again, only to repeat her puzzled lament after several more minutes of contemplative silence. After Mickey's death, Mary recalled this behavior with a laugh, a sort of fond perplexity about what was going on there. Despite the humorous turn she gave it, the tale of Kathryn's repeated hushed elegies was the only story Mary told from those dark days. Something in Kathryn's action was a touchstone for her, encapsulating the nature of the vigil and its grief. "I don't know." No questions or answers, no explanations and no demands. Only presence, faithfulness, and honesty.

During this period of watchful waiting, I left town for a long-planned weekend in New York City. I was anxious about leaving Mickey but decided to handle my concern by calling the P.I.C.U. each morning to talk with her parents. Saturday morning it was Mary who came to the phone. She told me that the evening before, when it was just Mary and Mickey in the room, Mickey had asked, "Am I going to die?"

"What did you say, Mary?"

"Well, jeez, I mean, what do you say? I said I hoped not, that we were trying to keep that from happening. But that, whatever was happening, we were going to be right there with her. No matter what, we're in this together."

"Good, good. So, what did she say then?"

"Nothing really. Just like 'okay,' and then she went back to sleep."

We talked a bit more, then I hung up and went on with a day of museums and theater, pleased that Mickey had been able to ask the question and that Mary had been able to allow it, without veering away, and to tell her what I thought was most important: that she would not be alone. I wondered whether, had Mickey asked me, I could have been honest (and brave) enough to say simply "Yes," and whether or not that reply would have been a better way to respond to this particular twelve-year-old. I was glad Mary had been the one she asked.

I called again Sunday morning, and this time it was Marshall who came to the phone. "Dr. Mohrmann, Mickey asked me something just now, and I don't know if I said the right thing."

"What was it?"

"She asked me if she was gonna die. And I just said, 'No way, Mick. Don't think about stuff like that. You just think about getting better.' I couldn't tell her the truth, Dr. Mohrmann. Did I do the right thing?"

"Sure," I said, "if that's what you were comfortable telling her." How could I chastise this heartbroken man? How could I ask him to say to his daughter what he could scarcely admit to himself? Besides, how do I know his answer was not just right, exactly what Mickey expected and wanted from her dad?

When I returned from that weekend I started agitating in earnest not only to end the isolation but to transfer Mickey out of the P.I.C.U. and back to her old room, which had been kept for her, cards still on the walls (fortunately, her bed had not been needed). Mickey's constant theme since entering the P.I.C.U. had been her desire to return to that room. Each time she roused from sleep, she asked the same question: "Why can't I go back to my room? I don't like this room. All my stuff is up there. I want to go back."

I could speculate about what a move back to her old room might mean to her. It contained as much of home as she could take with her, so it was as close to home as she could get. Plus, she had been in the hospital long enough to have learned the pediatric patients' conventional wisdom: a kid who gets "transferred to the P.I.C.U." never comes back—it's just the way adults get around telling us that that kid died. So if going to the P.I.C.U. is the euphemism for death, perhaps being transferred back to one's old room means survival. Or maybe Mickey just needed to yearn for something potentially attainable, knowing that her deepest wishes would not be granted.

The P.I.C.U. nurses said they would be willing to check in on her and supplement the floor nursing staff if her care became too much for them; the floor nurses wanted her back. Even with that, it took days of diplomacy and pleading, but finally all agreed that Mickey could be moved back to her old room, without isolation precautions. We all acknowledged that she was dying, that her death would come soon, that there was nothing more to be done by way of treatment and nothing to be gained by continuing intensive care.

She greeted the news of her impending move with as much enthusiasm as she could manage: "Good." That single syllable, spoken with the old asperity directed at those whose mental processors did not work as rapidly or precisely as hers, reminded us of who this child was, of the Mickey who was still there, still inhabiting the wracked body rapidly moving toward its end. She was awake for the move and, like a queen on her throne, received graciously the warm farewells of the P.I.C.U. staff and the welcoming embrace of the floor nurses. Once she was installed in her room, her parents pointed out to her that all the old decorations were still in place, envisioning them for her, assuring her that this was indeed the same old, familiar place. Mickey was home, such as it was. She broke into a broad grin, turned on her side, and fell deeply asleep.

Her parents and I watched her sleeping and spoke briefly, hesitantly of what we believed to be true, that Mickey would surely die soon, perhaps even that night or tomorrow—perhaps assisted on her way by her victory over pediatric protocol, by being the one kid who actually came back from the P.I.C.U. Her parents agreed: "This is where she should be. We won't be going back to the P.I.C.U., will we?"

"No," I said, "we won't. This is it."

It was now early evening, and I was not on call. I left and went home. I felt certain Mickey would die that night, but I had no official role on the team, and, for all my feelings of closeness to her parents, I was not so much part of her family that I should stay the night there. I was at a loss about where I should be, what I should do, even who I was now. I had done my final doctor act for Mickey by getting her transferred. What could my role be now? I knew nothing else to do but go home. Driving the thirty minutes to my apartment with a painful weight in my chest, I felt I was running away from something, something unfinished, undone, but I could not grasp what it might be. I was somehow failing to measure up but could not fathom what the missed standard might be. I knew only that I felt bad, really bad. The idea that this might be what grief is like did not occur to me.

At home I changed into more relaxed clothes, fixed and ate dinner, and watched television. Then the phone rang. It was the resident on call. Mickey had arrested. The team had resuscitated her, moved her back to the P.I.C.U., and hooked her up to a ventilator. "You *what?*" I screamed—but I think that was in my head only. I think I actually said something more like, "Oh, gosh. I'm on my way."

A thirty-minute drive back to the hospital—thirty minutes in which to deal with the turmoil of questions in my head. Why had I not stayed? Why had they resuscitated her? Why had I not foreseen this? I knew my colleagues. I knew that was what they would do. I just had not put it all together, had not imagined what the night would be like, what would actually happen when Mickey stopped breathing. And, I realized with sickening suddenness, I had never talked explicitly with the residents on call about how Mickey's parents and I understood the significance of her move out of the P.I.C.U. I had not said to them, "We think she'll die tonight, and if not tonight, very soon. She's ready; they're ready. When she dies, let her go. It's time. Let it happen here, in this room, with her parents here with her." I did not say it. Truth to tell, I did not think it, not that clearly. I had indeed left something undone.

Matt, the senior resident on call that night, met me at the entrance to the P.I.C.U. "She's gone," he said. "She arrested again and we couldn't get her back."

"Yes," I thought, "good. It's over. Finally. Good, Mick, good." What I said was, "Where is she?"

"There." Matt gestured toward the door of her old P.I.C.U. room, the one she had triumphantly sailed out of just a few hours before. "Her parents are back in the conference room. Curtis was on tonight too and happened to be up here seeing another patient when we were working on her. He knows them. He's in there with them." Curtis was the resident who had admitted Mickey the first time, back in April, and cared for her until I took over in May. He had never failed to ask about her when he saw me. I was glad he was there, someone they knew and knew cared about Mickey.

As I turned to go into the room to see her, Matt put his hand on my arm. "Wait a minute. Why don't you just take a minute to deal with this before you go in there." He said it with real concern, but I bristled at what I read as a patronizing tone, with the implication that I was less than professional, that I had crossed that bright line, dear to those who think they can see where it is, between caring about my patients and being over-involved with them.

"I'm fine," I said abruptly. "I want to see her, and then I'll go talk with her parents." He shrugged and turned away.

"Why did you do it, Matt?" I asked of his departing back. "You knew she was going to die. Why the code?"

"Every patient deserves our best efforts, Margaret," he said over his shoulder. "Of course we had to do it. We didn't even consider not doing it." He walked away.

I closed my eyes a moment, feeling the grief wash over me—grief at Mickey's death, certainly, but also grief that I had failed her and her parents at this most critical moment and left her in the hands of those who saw her only as Everypatient, not as beautiful, irreplaceable, dying Mick who needed to leave.

I entered her room—the room she had so wanted to be shut of—and saw her body lying on the bed, surrounded by the familiar detritus of a failed code. The board still under her torso; ripped-open packages of gauze, syringes, tubing scattered on the floor; the "crash cart" gaping open, standing at an angle to her bed. It was the kind of scene I had walked away from many times before. I knew what the room had been like a half-hour before when it was a live-action drama. I could imagine the clipped orders, the barked questions—"Can you get a pulse? Stop a minute and let me listen! How long has it been? Haven't you got that line in yet? Give me another epi!"—bouncing off the ugly tile walls that had been the last thing Mickey's eyes ever gazed upon.

The silence now was ripe and heavy. I walked over to the bed and gazed down at her. The endotracheal tube that had connected her to the ventilator was still in place, its anchoring tape obscuring much of her lower face. Her naked body was arrayed as it had been left, arms out to receive intravenous lines, disregarding her twelve-year-old girl's modesty, which she had emphatically taught me to honor months before when I had performed her first (and last) rectal exam. I arranged the tangled sheet as well as I could without removing the equipment from the bed, but I could only get it up to her waist. I caressed her bald head, told her goodbye, and left the room.

I walked slowly down to the conference room to see Mickey's parents. They were seated facing each other, with Curtis squatting in the space between, a hand reached out to each of them. I eased in quietly. Mary, facing the doorway by which I stood, kept her head down, weeping. Marshall's back was to me, his head bowed. As I walked around him, I put my hand on his shoulder. He jumped up and hugged me, crying, "She did it, Dr. Mohrmann. She beat 'em." He crumpled back into his chair, face in his hands. I reached over to Mary, who just nodded and grasped my hand. Then I sat in the chair between them.

"Dr. Evans here has been wonderful," Mary said, as she got control of her voice. "He knew Mickey from the beginning, you know, and he's here tonight."

I nodded my appreciation to Curtis, whose brimming eyes mirrored my own.

Then Marshall grabbed my hand, needing to explain. "We tried to tell 'em, Dr. Mohrmann. We knew she was going to die. She didn't want to leave her room. We tried to tell 'em it was all right, but they did it anyway. They brought her back down here and did all that stuff to her. And the whole time they were working on her, I sat there in that waiting room, saying 'Beat 'em, Mick! Beat 'em!' And she did!"

Thus the grieving father, forced to cheer on his daughter's death, pleading for absolution—"We tried to tell 'em! We tried!"—for having failed to protect her from this last insult, and asking it of me, who felt the same sense of failure and did not know how to separate it from grief for the loss of Mickey. Mary, the one who had always had so much more to say, was now the silent one, locked in a world of loss, ready to leave this place she hated.

At their request, I followed Mary and Marshall to their house, where Chris was waiting, keeping solitary vigil. Joey and Jenny were spending the night with Flo and Joe, but Chris had refused to leave the house, insisting on being dealt with as an adult in this crisis. They told him the news; he ducked his head and nodded, let himself be hugged, then got in the car with all of us to drive over to his grandparents. They knew when they saw us at the door. We tiptoed through the dining room where the children lay on cots—supposedly asleep, but I was unconvinced—to the kitchen, where we sat around the table and talked aimlessly. I do not remember whether we talked about the events of that evening or about Mickey herself or about necessary plans. I recall periods of silence and staring; attempts to take care of Chris, whose red-rimmed eyes belied his stoic demeanor; and studious ignoring of Joey and Jenny, lying prone on their cots on either side of the kitchen door, just outside the ring of light over the table, their heads propped up on their hands, eyes wide, staring solemnly back at me each time I glanced their way.

When we left after an hour or so, the children slept, or feigned sleep, once more, so we again tiptoed our way across the floor. They offered me a room for the night, but I insisted on returning to the hospital. I felt some need to be there; it was more my home than my apartment was. Back at the hospital, I determinedly set about taking down the cards from the walls of Mickey's room, packing them away with the stuffed animals and other souvenirs of home to return to her parents.

A few days later I went to the wake at the funeral home and the following day, along with some of the nurses who knew Mickey well, to the funeral at the family's parish church. At the wake, there were little cards of remembrance in the room, each with a poem about God's tendency to pluck the fairest flowers from Earth to beautify a heavenly garden. When I walked over to speak to the family, I could see that the casket was open. Flo immediately began urging me to go over and see how good Mickey looked. I resisted. Although open caskets are the practice in my own family, and I had not shied away from them before, this time I did not think I wanted to see her rehabilitated but dead face. However, by the time I was ready to leave, I realized how important it was to Flo, and possibly to Mary, that I pay my respects, so I went over to the casket and knelt on the prie-dieu set up in front of it. Out of the corner of my eye, I could see Flo nudge Mary and point to me, a smile of pleased satisfaction on her face. Mickey looked remarkably well, remarkably like the child I had first met in May, before the real tortures had begun. She was wearing the wig she had sported all summer. I remember, Mickey.

Chapter 5

Another Kind of Courage

PERHAPS NO OTHER DEATH, save Mickey's, during these early years so moved me as Luke's. Above all, Luke's death, which happened toward the end of my final year of residency, forced me to pay attention not only to the extraordinary courage some children display but also to the extraordinary demands we sometimes place on their small shoulders. I can still see in vivid detail the final scene of his story.

Luke was a nine-year-old boy in the terminal stage of cystic fibrosis. I had met him several times during my years at Hopkins, when he had been admitted for bouts of pneumonia. He had never been my patient, but I had covered for his doctor when he was off duty. I had been charmed by Luke's wit and directness. He was an acknowledged leader for the other children on the ward, full of a wonderful combination of good humor and no nonsense. The nurses adored him. His mother was in and out; she worked full-time and came for a few hours most evenings (his father was long out of the picture). She had little to say to the staff, just sat with Luke a bit, then left. She and Luke seemed to be on comfortable but not overly affectionate terms, asking little of each other, or so I thought.

This time I was on the ward as one of two senior residents. Luke was not assigned to my team, but he was covered by us on our call nights. The senior resident supervising the other team happened to be the doctor who had cared for him for the past two years. He told us that Luke was going to die this time. His lungs were ravaged by the disease; this latest infection was certainly the one that would finally tip him over. His doctor had exhausted the existing procedures used to wash the clogging mucus out of his airways, as well as cutting edge antibiotics used at dangerous-edge doses. Lung transplants were far in the future, unattainable. Luke was now expending great effort to breathe, gasping oxygen, unable to lie down flat in his bed.

All had been explained to his mother in great detail. In fact, when it had become apparent over the past year that Luke's condition was rapidly deteriorating and was sure to result in his death long before he reached adolescence, his mother was told many times about the absence of treatment options and what to expect over the next months. According to Luke's doctor, she had usually listened quietly, asking nothing, adding nothing, nodding in understanding if not in agreement. At the time of this hospitalization, she had been told with certainty that Luke would die this time, that there was no hope for another discharge home, however short. And this time she had spoken. She said no: this was not going to happen to her child. We would see, she had said. We would see that Luke would pull through this time and every other time. He was not going to leave her alone. Period.

When Luke's doctor had wanted to give him morphine to ease his constant air hunger and allow him some comfort and rest—and had to admit that doing so could hasten his death by diminishing his respiratory drive—she had refused to allow it. Luke was spending his last days sitting up in his bed, hunched forward over the bed table, oxygen prongs in his nose, heaving air in and out of his thin, bony chest and what remained of his thick, stiff lungs. He had no energy left for communication beyond a raised finger, an arched eyebrow.

Late one night, when I was on call, I sat with a couple of nurses at the big table in the nurses' station. Edie was the nurse responsible for Luke that night; in fact, she was always Luke's nurse when he was in the hospital. She knew him well and loved him dearly, and he obviously adored her. Edie shook her head sadly as she told me what had happened an hour or so earlier. She had gone in to check on Luke and found him sitting up, puffing away as usual, but his oxygen tubing and nasal prongs were lying on the bed beside him, aerating the bed clothes. Quietly, so as not to wake his mother who now, having heard the dire predictions, spent each night on a cot in his room, Edie replaced the prongs in his nose. Luke rolled his eyes up at her as she did so and rasped, with unmistakable sarcasm, "Thanks a lot!"

I shook my head with her. We agreed that Luke was ready to go. We believed that he knew there was no end for this suffering but *the end* and wanted to get on with it, whether his mother was ready or not. "I'm sorry," I said to her. "How hard." She nodded and turned to the intercom system on the wall to check on him yet again. Luke's breathing was so stertorous that it was easy to hear him when the speaker system from his bed to the nurses' station was activated. Edie flipped the switch, and we heard nothing.

We jumped up and went the few steps to his room, which was just across from the nurses' station. Luke was not in his bed. The oxygen tubing was hissing into the sheet, the IV apparatus dangling from the pole. His mother was still asleep on her cot. I opened the door to the bathroom, a few feet from his bed, and there was Luke, facedown on the floor. I picked up his small, wasted body, moving him far enough into the room to check his pulses, putting my stethoscope on his chest. No heartbeat, no respiratory effort. Luke was dead.

Edie and I looked at each other and then, without saying a word, together gathered him up from the floor and placed him back on his bed. I reattached the IV to the catheter in his arm while she turned off the oxygen at the wall. We drew the covers up to his chest and stood for a moment, each of us holding one of his hands. Edie looked up at me and cut her eyes silently toward the sleeping figure in the corner. I took a deep breath, nodded, walked over to the cot, and touched Luke's mother on the shoulder.

"Mrs. Lorenzo, Mrs. Lorenzo. I'm sorry to wake you."

"What? What is it?" She raised herself partway up, shaking her head to clear it.

"Luke just died, Mrs. Lorenzo. I'm so sorry."

"Oh. Oh. Just now?"

"Yes. Very quietly. He just stopped."

Brave Luke, taking care of her even at the end, even as he took care of himself.

PART II

Accompanying

Attend: II. To watch over, wait upon (with service), accompany as a servant, go with, be present at
—To apply oneself to the care or service of (a person), esp. to watch over and wait upon, to minister to (the sick)
—To follow, escort, or accompany, for the purpose of rendering services

She can do nothing for the parts irreparably lost. But she has something to leave in the dark reaches, the space in each one where the earliest, inviolable fable of self still stands intact, ready to respond. . . . She can plant a start in that place waiting to be proved wrong, a plot that will still heal at the first touch of fresh, outrageously naïve narrative.

—Richard Powers, *Operation Wandering Soul*

The stories in part II have lost some of the frayed edge of inexperience and unreflective reaction that characterize many of the preceding narratives in which I am often just trying to hold it together from one situation to the next. Although the business of shepherding children and parents through a critical or chronic illness is clearly something I am still in the process of learning in the following stories, my voice in these tales becomes more thoughtful, saying more about what is going on rather than simply reporting what happened. I am perhaps somewhat more balanced in my level of involvement with patients and families; the variations of distance are more likely to be related to the duration of the relationship than to unevenness in the intensity of my engagement.

I struggle here with other tasks related to being the attending: being not only a good doctor for my patients but also a good colleague for my fellow faculty physicians and the nurses with whom I work, as well as a good teacher and model for our trainees. You will notice little mention in these stories of students or residents, although they were present and involved in some fashion in every tale. In general, however, they did not accompany me when I spoke with parents, when difficult decision making, the breaking of terrible news, or simply the deepening of acquaintance was the task. At first, this was because I did not invite them to come along; I was too unsure of myself in those crucial negotiations to welcome a witness who might learn a wrong lesson or, worse, find the teacher inadequate. When I became more confident and asked trainees to participate in conferences with parents, they almost always refused: I'm too busy, that's the attending's job, I'd be too uncomfortable. I did not know then how to overcome their resistance nor how to say, clearly and convincingly, what there was to be learned and how important the lessons were for their education in doctoring. Perhaps this book can be part of my belated explanation, for them and for me.

The fact of death and the telling of it to family members had loomed large for me during my residency, as I believe it does for most physicians in training. Only later did I begin to fathom what these wrenching episodes were teaching me about being a doctor. Times of participation in a patient's dying can be periods of concentrated and difficult learning, when the strands of intellectual and emotional engagement in a "case" collapse together into a node of intense activity that then slows to a full and intimate stillness. At that finally quiet place, I learned that a doctor always has two basic choices. Each option has a number of possible variations, but the fundamental decision remains binary. One is to run away, mentally if not physically, to shy away from the bare truth of loss, the intimations of inadequacy, the grief or anger, or sometimes hardest to bear, the gratitude of those bereft. The other option is to stay, mentally as well as physically, and to remain open to what is there to be known and felt, open to being moved and thereby changed into a physician who now understands better what is asked of him or her.

The children I cared for in my resident years and their families determined which of these two options I would end up choosing. They held me fast, compelling my attention long enough for me to begin learning the signal necessity of remaining present and allowing myself to be moved if I wished to mature into the sort of doctor my patients needed me to be and, for that matter, if I wished to foster my own emotional growth and well-being. After my residency, the years I spent directing a P.I.C.U. confirmed and continued that teaching as I was confronted with death or its imminent possibility with daunting regularity.

What I learned—or rather how I was formed in the P.I.C.U.—by staying beside children as they died, staying with parents as they wept or raged, as they watched the monitors mark the last heartbeats taught me also how to accompany the children who lived—those who survived a severe acute illness, those whose disorders were lingering and interminable, even those who never got that sick and their parents. The obligation for the attending physician to be present, to walk alongside, is no less important when patients are facing the dilemmas of living than when they are confronting the distresses of dying.

Chapter 6

※ ———————— ※

Being There

> ※ **Keith**

A SLIM, LONG-LIMBED thirteen-year-old, with smooth, dark brown skin and close-cropped hair, Keith was just coming into his adult body. He had gone to the beach one morning with his older sister and her children, and while he was there, he had developed a headache and complained about it enough that his sister had packed up the kids and headed for home. In the car he began banging his head against the side window because it hurt so much. His sister made a rapid detour and brought him directly to the emergency room. A brief examination was enough to convince the medical staff that this was more than a migraine.

Keith, still fully conscious and complaining bitterly of the pain in his head, was quickly brought over to the main hospital to have his head scanned on the way to the pediatric ward, where he was to be admitted for close observation and evaluation. By the time he reached the scan some fifteen minutes later, he was comatose. During the scan, he stopped breathing. The doctors present—one had accompanied him from the emergency room, others were there waiting for him—immediately re-suscitated him, placed him on ventilatory support, and rolled him up to the P.I.C.U.

Enough of a scan had been obtained by that time to show a huge cyst deep in his brain. It appeared to have expanded suddenly, and to devastating effect, probably because of bleeding into it. The neurosurgeons took one look at the image and at Keith and shook their heads; there was no way to get in there and fix this. When I first examined Keith upon his arrival in the P.I.C.U., he already met neurologic criteria for brain death. We went through the necessary protocols of time and testing and consultation, but he never regained any signs that suggested anything other than a verdict of brain death. Forty-eight hours after his headache started, I pronounced him dead.

Keith's mother was an older woman, in her midfifties, a widow, and Keith was her youngest child. She had several older children, all adults living in homes of their own, some far away. Keith had been the only child at home for some years now. She said he was a "good boy," an obedient boy, who liked being with his mama and behaved well in school and made good grades. Some of his older siblings had gone to college, and Keith was determined that he would too. She was at a loss to comprehend this lightning strike—who would not be? He was fine when he left her that morning to go to the beach. No, he had not complained of any headaches before. No, there had not been anything out of the ordinary, just a happy thirteen-year-old heading off for an outing with the little nieces and nephews he so enjoyed. How could this be? I had no answers for that, none at all.

During the two days required to confirm the diagnosis of brain death, I sat with her often, sometimes at her request explaining his condition again and why it took this long to be sure, sometimes listening to her deeper questions and her grief. Mostly she was silent, waiting, and I was silent with her. Late in the afternoon of the second day, our vigil ended when I told her Keith was definitely dead, that all the tests had continued to confirm that the tumor's pressure had destroyed the parts of his brain necessary to keep him alive and that I was now going to take him off the artificial support. She said she would like to sit with him after I did that.

Back in the P.I.C.U., the nurses put a rocking chair by Keith's bed for her. I turned off the ventilator and detached it from the tube that went into his windpipe. A nurse removed his intravenous lines. We cleared the bed of debris and pulled the sheet halfway up his chest, leaving his arms uncovered. He looked so healthy—beautiful, really—like a young man asleep, or sunbathing perhaps, his body unmarked by trauma or age. But he did not breathe, and the look of death was unmistakable.

I went back to get his mother and brought her in, leaning on my arm, to sit by her son. She lowered herself into the rocking chair, picked up his hand, and stroked it. She gazed long and hard at his face in repose, perhaps seeking some answer to her impossible questions, some message to respond to her despair. Then she carefully placed his hand back by his side and leaned back in the chair, still looking at his face. Slowly she began to rock and, as her rocking motions gradually increased in amplitude before settling into a steady rhythm, so did her low-voiced keening. It began as a sort of humming murmur, as though she were singing an old lullaby of comfort for him, for herself.

As she rocked, her music became a little louder and began to break up into sounds more like speech, a sort of hushed chant or muffled glossolalia. Then the tongues of her sorrow fused into one intelligible language as she found voice to articulate her grief. Still rocking, she turned her face from her son to me where I stood at the foot of the bed, bearing mute witness, and said what she had discovered about the contours of her loss: "Who's going to sit on the porch in the evening with me? Who's going to go to the grocery store with me?"

I looked back, my tears mirroring hers, but I had no answer. I nodded in time with her rocking, feeling my sorrow for her loss. We stayed for a long moment, gazing and nodding at each other, as though agreeing that this, indeed, is grief. Then she expelled a long sigh, brought her chair to a still point, and turned back to look once more at her son. She pushed herself up out of the chair, stood a moment completing her gaze— perhaps imprinting his face with finality on her memory—turned, nodded to me, and left the room without looking back.

By the time I knew Keith and his mother, I had learned (the hard way, mostly) what was being asked of me at the time of a patient's death. I knew enough now to stay and be silent, to absorb what was happening, and to meet it with unguarded openness, a willingness to be moved. But it is Keith's mother and the scene beside her son's deathbed that I recall when I am asked what I learn, besides the importance of being there to support the family, or how and in what way I am changed by being fully present at such moments. Standing at the foot of Keith's bed, attending to his mother, I comprehended—immediately and indelibly—the face and texture and grip of grief, the posture of a life already haunted by the shadow of one who has left first and too soon. Pediatricians are often taught that the death of a child strikes so deeply because of the loss of the parents' anticipated future. There is much truth to that, but Keith's mother reminds me of the enormity of the pain of also losing present joy and treasured companionship. I hope for Keith's mother that having someone to say it to, someone there to receive and hold the wrenching articulation of her sorrow, was the beginning of living with the loss, a first step toward whatever healing could be.

≳ Tom and Ellie

EARLY ONE MIDWINTER EVENING, I was asked to admit two children at once to the P.I.C.U., two children from the same family. There had been a house fire, and the children and their mother had been carried from the house by firefighters. The mother was on her way to another hospital to have her burns and smoke inhalation treated, and she was expected to survive. The children, however, were not breathing when they were brought out of the house, covered in soot and apparently untouched by the flames. They were resuscitated on the front lawn of the house by firefighters and emergency medical personnel. The temperature outside was about twenty degrees, and the resuscitative efforts had taken more than thirty minutes. The children continued to require artificial ventilation as they were brought to the medical center.

They filled the P.I.C.U. with the smell of wood smoke. Their sooty bodies required several sponge baths before they were fully clean, and we could then see how much they resembled each other, their raggedly cut, thin blonde hair spread out around their now pasty white faces. Two-year-old Ellie and her four-year-old brother Tom had body temperatures in the low eighties, at least fifteen degrees below normal, when they arrived. They showed no signs of brain activity, but our fervent hope was that the hypothermia had protected them from the worst effects of the oxygen deprivation caused by the smoke and their subsequent arrests. We knew that the hope was tenuous, that they had suffered from low oxygen long enough to make their hearts stop and that the oxygenless period had occurred in the warmth of a burning house, but hope we did. We rewarmed them slowly and carefully—warm intravenous fluids and heated liquids down tubes into their stomachs, in addition to blankets and heating lamps—gradually letting their core temperatures rise to normal over several hours, in order to avoid the damage that can result from rewarming that is either too rapid or too unbalanced (which happens when skin warms faster than internal organs, thus shifting blood flow away from vital centers—brain, kidneys, heart—into newly expanded blood vessels in the warm skin).

Once the children's body temperatures were back to normal, we tested their brain functions thoroughly and found that each of them still fit the criteria for brain death. Their lungs were surprisingly healthy after all that smoke, suggesting they had not breathed for long inside the burning house; evidence of smoke damage on their chest X rays cleared quickly. Nevertheless, the oxygen deprivation had done its work. Tom and Ellie would not survive.

I explained the situation to their father over the telephone. He had checked in frequently by phone to see if there was any change in the children's condition but had stayed by their mother's side as she received treatment for her injuries. She had some significant burns, especially on one arm, and was still coughing up the effects of the smoke, but she would be able to leave the hospital in a day or so. He understood and accepted, tearfully, the confirmation of brain death when it came but asked if we could keep the children on the ventilators until his wife could come see them. She would be there within forty-eight hours, he was sure. Of course we could, I said, although I cautioned him that it would be difficult to sustain their bodies—or justify holding their places in the small, always-full P.I.C.U.—much longer than that.

The next morning he called the P.I.C.U. to say that his wife had been discharged and that they were on their way over. They had decided that they wanted the children to be baptized while they were still "alive" on the ventilators. Baptism was something they had never gotten around to doing, their father said, always thinking there was plenty of time for that when they were older and could say for themselves whether they wanted it. The family did not belong to a church and had no particular clergyperson in mind. I asked if they had a denominational preference and assured him we would find a pastor to do the baptisms. One of the P.I.C.U. nurses knew the clergyman of a church in the parents' preferred denomination who had often been called upon to act as unofficial chaplain for patients of his tradition. The nurse called him with our request, and he readily agreed to come.

Early that afternoon, the children's parents arrived. Their mother looked drawn and weary, holding her bandaged arm to her chest, their father grim and silent. I talked with them about what to expect in the P.I.C.U., how the children looked, what the tubes and monitors meant. They had little to say, receiving the information dully, dazed by the events of the past few days and their anticipation of what the next hour would hold. They came into the unit, clutching each other for support, and at first stood together by the bed of each child in turn, touching a hand, kissing a cheek, smoothing hair, murmuring words of love and apology and farewell. The children's beds were diagonally across from each other, abutting opposite walls of the small room (the particular needs of the other two patients in the room had made it impossible to place Tom and Ellie side by side), so their parents could not physically attend to both children at once. They moved back and forth, together and separately, for a last touch, a final memory.

The pastor had arrived. When it seemed the right time, I asked if they wanted to talk with him before the baptism. "No," their father said abruptly, choking on his words. "Let's just do it."

I escorted the pastor into the P.I.C.U. and introduced him to the parents and to the children. He spoke briefly, softly with the parents in one corner of the room. Then we—the pastor, the children's parents, the nurses, and I—moved first to Tom's bed. The rite was brief; the pastor included a prayer appropriate for a death. We then silently moved to Ellie's bedside and repeated the ceremony. When the pastor was finished, the parents shook his hand and thanked him, then looked up at me questioningly.

"What happens now?"

"I take them off the ventilators. Their hearts will slow down and stop. Then we'll wrap them up snugly and take them to the hospital morgue. After the autopsies, which should be done later today, the funeral home will come get them."

We had already discussed the arrangements, the name of the funeral home, and they had given permission for the children's bodies to be autopsied, wanting, they said, some good to come out of all this. They nodded, thanked me and the nurses, and left. They had told me they did not want to be there when the ventilators were stopped, nor did they want to see the children "cold and dead," as they put it.

When they left, the nurses and I spent a few minutes in our own silent rituals of grieving and of honoring the children—touching them, straightening their bedclothes, supporting each other. I turned off the ventilators and detached the tubing, first from Tom—in order of his age and his baptism—and then from Ellie, and then I helped the nurses prepare their bodies for the morgue attendant to take them away. I wrote the "death note" in their charts and filled out the death certificates the morgue attendant brought with him. Then I returned to my office and sat quietly for a while, letting myself feel the full weight of their deaths.

I checked in on my other patients and went home for the night. The next morning I realized that my home phone had not rung at all during the night. This was quite unusual, because the residents routinely called me about every admittance to my service or with questions about our patients, and we had several patients in the hospital whose conditions were far from stable. Still puzzling over this odd absence, I mentioned it to the chief resident after morning rounds.

"Oh," she said cheerily. "I can explain that. I knew you'd be upset after having to take those two kids off their ventilators yesterday, so I told everyone to call me with their questions to sort of give you some time away from it all."

I was so angry, I'm not sure what I said in reply, whether I let her know the extent of my displeasure. My immediate reaction, I think, had to do primarily with the tacit presumption of weakness, of some sort of emotional fragility that her patronizing decision imputed to me and relayed to the rest of the residents. Maybe she thought I just couldn't take it, or she decided I needed to fall apart and, while falling apart, would not be able to do my job well. She was way out of line. And how embarrassing! How was I to correct the impression of me she had created for the house staff? Beyond my anger and discomfiture, however, I was more puzzled than ever. Why would she think I needed that kind of care? I knew quite well that I had been distressed, that I had dealt with it, and that I needed no "time away" in order to recover—which put another slant on the question: Why didn't I need recovery time?

It has taken me years to understand at any depth why I was so sure that her actions were not just condescending (and a blow to my pride) but wrong-headed, that in her entirely well-intentioned effort to take care of me she had done precisely the wrong thing. I had been fully present for the tragedy played out in the P.I.C.U. that day, a participant in the poignant baptismal rites, a witness to the parents' farewells. I was the one who wrote the orders to take the children off their ventilators, and I was the one who physically carried out those orders. I had allowed myself to feel the pain of those two deaths, and I had spent time afterward just sitting with it, letting it be real, letting Tom and Ellie and their ends matter to me. That was what I needed to do to honor their short lives and to honor myself in this difficult job.

I believe that it is by being present in such ways that I, and other doctors, find healing for the wounds that the practice of medicine inflicts on us. Being there fully, experiencing the awfulness directly without shielding myself by leaving (physically, mentally, or emotionally) gives me both clarity about who is actually suffering this terrible loss—the parents, in ways I can neither imagine nor vicariously undergo and to a degree that puts my sense of loss in appropriate perspective—and the opportunity to acknowledge and experience my own legitimate emotions. Having done that, I no longer have to expend energy needed for other parts of my job trying to keep at bay a grief I would not allow myself to admit.

I have often been asked how I could possibly do P.I.C.U. work, how I could "survive" it. My answer is that I survived—more than that, thrived on—the pain of being present for such heartbreaking events by being truly present and allowing my heart to *be* broken. The heart that can break, again and again, in the face of such suffering and grief becomes softer, more resilient, more capacious. After Tom and Ellie died I was ready to meet new patients, to handle queries about care, to be the more capable doctor I had become that day.

Chapter 7

Intensive Care

I HEARD ABOUT her days before I ever met her. Jennie Daugherty was an eleven-year-old girl who had become quite ill as the result of an ear infection. The infection had led to mastoiditis—infection of the porous bone located just behind the ear—and then, worse luck, to perforation of the mastoid bone and formation of an abscess between that part of her skull and her brain: the once-in-a-career reminder of why pediatricians take ear infections seriously. While on the way to the operating room to have the abscess drained, Jennie had stopped breathing. She was immediately resuscitated, and the surgical procedure had then been carried out successfully. Given what she had been through, I was told, Jennie was in remarkably good shape and recuperating in a room on the regular pediatrics ward: an interesting story to be mentally filed away for use as a minatory example for my lectures on otitis.

However, two days after the arrest and the operation, Jennie developed pneumonia. Her condition rapidly worsened to the point that she needed a bed in the P.I.C.U. because of her significant respiratory distress and need for oxygen; because her neurosurgical problems were no longer the issue, Jennie was transferred to my care. It soon became obvious that she required ventilatory support—her own efforts could not keep her sufficiently oxygenated nor could she long sustain such work—so she was sedated, intubated, and connected to a ventilator that did the work of breathing for her while we tried to figure out what was going on and why.

That day was the beginning of a long and arduous course in the P.I.C.U. for Jennie, her family, and our staff. It appeared that her lungs

had been attacked by an organism—based on blood analyses, we sus-
pected the culprit was the cytomegalovirus—which had taken advantage
of her weakened condition and of the damage that was likely to have
resulted from her arrest a couple of days before. The combination of in-
sults had led to her current problem: Adult Respiratory Distress Syndrome (A.R.D.S.), designated "adult" in order to distinguish it from
R.D.S., a pathophysiologically similar disorder found in premature newborns (the *A* in A.R.D.S. has more recently come to stand for "acute").

The problem in this disorder is loss (in premature babies, immature
development) of surfactant, a substance that normally lines the alveoli (air
sacs) of the lungs and keeps them open during exhalation so that they
remain slightly expanded even when the lungs have emptied. Without
surfactant, alveoli collapse as air leaves them, and collapsed alveoli, like
balloons that have never been inflated, are very difficult, sometimes impossible, to open up again, no matter how hard one tries to suck in air
or push it in with a ventilator. Alveoli are the sites at which oxygen in
inhaled air is transferred into the blood and the waste product of respiration—carbon dioxide—is released in exchange, then breathed out.
Without a sufficient number of functioning alveoli, respiration—the gas
exchange essential for life—cannot occur.

The primary object of artificial ventilation in A.R.D.S. is to provide
both an inflating pressure capable of opening collapsed alveoli and
enough residual pressure in the airways at the end of expiration to keep
the alveoli open for the next inspiration. Sometimes mechanical ventilation works, but other times the lung damage is so severe that large numbers of alveoli cannot be reopened or have been destroyed by oxygen
starvation or obliterated by the debris of infection, and there is no longer
an adequate surface remaining for the necessary exchange of gases. In that
case, no matter how forcefully and frequently air is pumped into the
lungs nor how much oxygen the air contains, blood oxygen levels stay
low or continue falling, and carbon dioxide levels rise, a situation that
cannot be survived for long.

Sometimes the ventilatory pressure, the force with which the oxygen-
rich air has to be pushed in, is too much for the lung tissue to handle,
especially the collapsed, inflamed, stiff areas, and the lung will tear at
those points of least flexibility, releasing air into the pleural cavity that

separates the lungs from the surrounding chest wall. This escaped air—termed a pneumothorax, air in the chest cavity where it does not belong—not only cannot get out but also expands in volume with each new inspired breath that whistles through the tear. The pneumothorax puts increasing counterpressure on the lung, acting to collapse it even as the ventilator tries to expand it, and can be relieved only by providing an exit for the bottled-up air. This is done by putting a tube through the chest wall into the air pocket to let the air escape and allow the lung to reinflate, if it will. Because of the overall inflexibility of the lungs in A.R.D.S. and the high pressures required to keep the alveoli inflated, it is a condition immensely complicated in its treatment by the frequent creation of pneumothoraces.

Once Jennie was on the ventilator, we soon recognized that she would indeed require inordinate pressures to get her blood oxygen levels up and carbon dioxide levels down into a livable range and keep them there. Over and over, we increased the pressure a bit and watched her oxygen levels rise gratifyingly, only to see them drift down again within hours, necessitating yet another bump in pressure—and so the cycle continued. All the while, we wondered when her first inevitable pneumothorax would appear; even healthy lung tissue, elastic as it is, would not tolerate the sorts of pressures we were forcing into her damaged lungs. We did not have to wait long. A dramatic plunge in her oxygen level, visible on her blue lips, signaled the presence of the rogue air pushing back against her struggling lungs. A pediatric surgeon inserted the chest tube between her ribs, into the pleural cavity, and with the escape of the trapped air came a pink flush to her lips as her oxygen levels climbed back toward normal. But that was only the first such event. Over the next several weeks, Jennie suffered multiple pneumothoraces; at one time, she had five chest tubes protruding from her thin, little girl's chest.

During those weeks her blood oxygen hovered at or below the lowest acceptable level. She would sometimes go for days with the level significantly lower than normal, and nothing we did to raise it made any difference. But somehow, all through that time, Jennie remained alert and engaged, intense brown eyes staring out from her pallid face, except during the brief periods of sedation necessary for the placement of yet another chest tube. Her blue lips would chatter on, despite the inconvenience of the tracheostomy—which had been placed after the first week of her illness, when we knew for certain that she was going to need ventilatory support for a long time—trying to communicate with us and with her family, and usually succeeding. We knew, because she told us over and over again, two important things about Jennie: she wanted to eat, and she wanted to go to Disney World when this was all over.

Eating was out of the question, not just eating by mouth, but even food placed into her stomach through a tube. The ventilatory pressures made the possibility of regurgitation from her stomach too likely, and aspiration of any foreign materials, whether forced up from her stomach or choked down during swallowing, would be the final straw for her sick lungs. So her "food" came to her entirely intravenously—nutritionally complete but not at all satisfying to unstimulated taste buds or empty stomach. Not surprisingly, Jennie developed a decided dislike of the lemon-flavored mouth swabs that were a poor substitute for a lollipop, much less for a hamburger. As for Disney World, her parents were ready to promise her the moon if she would just get better; Disney World was a cinch.

Mr. and Mrs. Daugherty were an older couple. Mr. Daugherty, retired after thirty years of teaching history in high school, and his wife ran a small appliance-repair business out of their home. After many years of trying and failing to conceive a child, they had adopted an infant, their now sixteen-year-old daughter, Anne. Jennie, appearing about five years later, was an unexpected conception, the pregnancy they thought they would never experience. They were devoted to both their children, overwhelmed by what was happening, and deeply reliant on their Christian faith to see them—and Jennie—through. They were warm and embracing, trusting and intelligent people, deferential to medical expertise, but also full of hope that God would not take this gift-child away from them. At our first encounter, they told me that there were already prayer groups "around the world" praying for Jennie. Their sense of universal and transcendental support and the determined optimism that sprang from it was something they alluded to often, especially on the many occasions when I had to admit that we had reached the far limits of what medical technology could do.

In the face of their persistent certainty that all would (and must) be well, I often found myself in the role of pessimist, emphasizing what I increasingly believed to be the case: Jennie could not survive this catastrophic illness. After three weeks of hammering away at her lungs, using every variety of ventilatory technology available, we still could not keep her oxygen levels up. Jennie, that skinny little preteen, displayed immense fortitude and endurance as she continued to chirrup away about Disney World and getting back to school, and we were impressed by her apparent cognitive perseverance in the face of such physiological ruin. But surely this could not continue, and I could see no way out; healing was fast becoming unimaginable. Thus, against the Daughertys' faith in the power of prayer and their pleasure at their daughter's alertness, I continually displayed the medical "facts" of the situation: Her lungs are no better; if anything, they're worse. This can't go on. I'm afraid I can't offer you much hope. I fear that we're going to see her oxygen levels drift down even farther, and we won't be able to bring them up. We're using maximal ventilatory assistance now. There's nowhere else to go if this doesn't work.

Anne was furious. "You're telling me my sister's going to die, and I just don't believe it. You're all wrong. She's going to be all right. I don't know why you keep telling us all this bad stuff. She's going to be all right."

To which all I could say, taking on what I thought to be the position of wisdom and experience, was, "We all hope you're right, Anne, we really do. It's just hard to see it that way right now."

Her reply was a "hmmpf," a glare, and tightly crossed arms. Her parents would make soothing noises toward her, which she ignored, and then nod to me, telling me that they understood—with tears slipping down their cheeks once again—and that they would stay here and keep on praying.

At some point in the fifth week of this arduous marathon, Jennie stopped getting worse. One by one the chest tubes were taken out, one every couple of days, and new ones were not needed. Her oxygen levels remained stable, without further increases in ventilatory pressure (not that we could have increased it; she had long since passed any reasonable limit on that measure). And then her oxygen levels began improving.

Slowly—excruciatingly slowly—we cut back on the pressures, and her oxygenation remained normal. Somehow, for some reason our science could not explain, Jennie was getting better.

It took several days before I could bring myself to acknowledge this to her parents and her sister. They already knew, of course; they were aware of every move we made on Jennie's behalf. They watched the tubes come out and stay out. They saw the pressure inching down and saw that Jennie was not dying as it all happened. They knew healing was afoot long before I was willing to admit it, to begin proffering real hope where before I had seen none. By the end of the sixth week, Jennie was off the ventilator, breathing room air (not oxygen-enriched) on her own, with normal blood oxygen levels. And she wanted to eat.

Next problem: how to feed a child who has been on parenteral nutrition for a month and a half and has undergone an assault on her body—mechanically and chemically, from inhuman pressures and long stretches of inadequate oxygen—that was likely to have injured, among other things, the lining of her intestines. The medical consensus: very slowly. Our nutrition consultants advised a progression of baby steps for reintroducing food to her gut. Jennie was ravenous. To her immense frustration, it took several days for her to advance from sips of water to bowls of gelatin and then, with great fanfare and rejoicing, to a plate of rice and baked chicken—real food, chewable, with (some) taste.

In accordance with the nutritionist's advice, for a couple of days she got chicken and rice at every meal, including breakfast. It did not take long for her to rebel, pushing the offending dish away, begging again for "real" food, different food. I sized her up, glowering in her bed, recalled that she had suffered no problems with anything she had eaten thus far, knew she needed to get out of the hospital before some other bug found her, and threw caution—and the nutritionist's advice—to the winds: "Order whatever you want from the menu. If you want your folks to bring you something from McDonald's, fine. Eat whatever you want. Let's see how you do."

She grinned and pointed to her father, who left immediately to return a half-hour later with a Big Mac, fries, and a milkshake. I shuddered at the thought of the lactose, the fat, and the red meat hitting her poor gut and wondered if I had been foolish—or worse, negligent—to give in to her whines. Too late, the deed was done. She did fine, with never a rumble from her "poor" and apparently also now happy and satisfied stomach.

Jennie went home soon after that. I made a few home visits over the next month or so to be sure she was continuing to do well. Within a year, her lung function tests returned to normal, another unexpected event. We had assumed she would be left with some degree of more or less problematic lung damage, from the high-pressure treatment if not from the disease itself, and be at significant lifelong risk of chronic lung disease, equivalent to that acquired from a multiyear history of smoking. But the follow-up evaluations suggested otherwise. Her lung function was not detectibly different from that of any other child her age who had had no respiratory disease. It seemed that the Daughertys' prayed-for miracle healing was complete.

Over the next several years, until I moved away, I was Jennie's pediatrician. Her parents were now even more attached to and protective of this daughter who had been given to them twice over. As Jennie entered adolescence, underlying family tensions and, doubtless, the lingering effects of the hospital experience took their toll. Jennie's unpredictable behavior and attitudes were an enigma to her parents; they were at a loss to account for or respond to her squalls of tears and angry recriminations. At the same time, I was concerned about her timidity outside the home and the diffuse anxiety that seemed to pervade her school and social life. I talked with them a number of times about psychological counseling, but Mr. and Mrs. Daugherty were very reluctant. They wrestled openly with their suspicion that secular therapy was in competition with or even incompatible with Christian belief. I urged them to consider the likelihood that Jennie's severe illness experience had engendered a degree of turmoil and fearfulness that would not go away on its own, while at the same time putting forward the possibility that God could work through therapists too.

They were mulling over my latest recommendation of a psychiatrist whose practice explicitly reflected her own Christian commitments when Jennie's behavior reached a crisis point. Mrs. Daugherty called me at home one Saturday morning: Jennie had locked herself in the bathroom with a kitchen knife, threatening to kill herself. While we were on the phone, Mrs. Daugherty provided a play-by-play narration of events as Mr. Daugherty convinced Jennie to unlock the door and disarmed her with little difficulty. But Jennie was still insisting that she wanted to die and would find a way to do it. She was not quite thirteen years old.

After talking with Jennie and her parents long enough to be sure she would be safe for the time being, I arranged for her to be seen by a psychiatrist that afternoon. As a result, she was admitted to an adolescent mental health facility. I was relieved at first, not only because she would be protected there from her suicidal urges but also because she would begin getting the therapy I had long wanted for her. Her parents were dismayed at the turn of events, but frightened enough by her threats to accept the need for hospitalization.

Unfortunately, this particular hospital may not have been the ideal place. The therapists decided from the start that Jennie's problem was her overprotective parents, as they told Mr. and Mrs. Daugherty. Consequently, after an initial meeting, the hospital staff kept Jennie's parents at arm's length, sharply limiting their contact with their daughter and refusing to talk further with them about her treatment or course. With her parents' permission, I offered to talk with her psychiatrist about her medical history and my knowledge of the family, but I was rebuffed; my calls went unanswered. The Daughertys called me frequently in their concern. I assured them that Jennie was in the right place and told myself that their anxiety reflected precisely their too-close attachment, but as the weeks passed and the therapists' wall remained in place, I became less willing to make excuses for their unprofessional and, I feared, untherapeutic approach. After a month of frustrated worry and increasingly frequent phone calls from Jennie begging to come home, her parents lost patience with the therapists and took Jennie out of the hospital. Whatever did or did not go on that month—I tend to think that, at best, it was not a particularly helpful experience for anyone—at least Jennie learned not to threaten suicide again. But I was not able to sell her or her parents on any sort of counseling after that experience, at least not until a much later crisis of a different sort forced the issue once again.

At fifteen, Jennie was still quite timid and retiring; she seemed a very young fifteen. On a routine visit, with her mother in the waiting room while I did Jennie's physical examination, I asked my usual questions about her social life. To my surprise, she shyly admitted she was dating someone steadily. He was a year older, a junior at her high school, and she knew he was the one she wanted to marry: "But we're going to wait until I finish school, of course." Then, in reply to my next necessary question and after a long, head-down hesitation, she told me they had been having intercourse for some months now.

"Are you using any kind of birth control, Jennie?"

"No! I don't need to."

"Why not?" I asked, genuinely puzzled.

"Well, you remember when I was so sick when I was little?" Oh, yes, I remember. "They told me that my ovaries were damaged, and I would never be able to have babies. So, we don't need to use any birth control." She looked up at me innocently, no hint of doubt or guile on her face.

I could not begin to fathom who "they" might be, but that was not the most important issue here. "That's not true, Jennie. There's no reason to think that your ovaries have anything at all wrong with them, no reason to think you can't have babies."

"Oh," she whispered, her hand over her shocked mouth. "Oh."

Oh, where to begin. This child is not ready for a sexual relationship, much less for babies. I asked her about her decision to have sex, and as I expected, her answer was all about pleasing the boyfriend she was so happy to have.

"Do you like it, Jennie?"

"Oh, yes. Well, not as much as he does, but I love being so close to him, you know? He's really good to me, he doesn't force me or anything, but I know it's really important to him."

The first form of birth control I discussed with her was abstinence. This was immediately rejected because, as she told me with solemn fervor, "But Dr. Mohrmann, I *neeeed* it." Yes, well . . .

I shall take a moment here to congratulate myself for not laughing out loud. She was so earnest, so sure, so, well, needy, that there did not seem to be any way then (if there ever is) to explore other reasons for that need or other ways to satisfy it, much less to introduce the notion of unfillable needs. Jennie was adamant that her mother not know about this, and I was adamant that she not become pregnant, so we worked out a way to keep her supplied with birth control pills without her parents' knowledge. It was far from an ideal solution, but it seemed the best one open to us. A few months later she called one afternoon to tell me, with a sort of nonchalance, that she had stopped taking the pills because she had broken up with that boyfriend and had decided that sex was not for her just now. Good, Jen. Keep me posted.

About a year later, I got a call at home from Jennie one rainy Friday evening. She was oddly inarticulate, and it did not take long to realize why. She was drunk and in a panic. With a lot of pressing, I was able to piece together the story. She was at home; her parents were out of town for the night, her sister at college. When her current boyfriend came to pick her up for their date, they decided to take advantage of her unwonted freedom by having a drink or two from her parents' lone bottle of vodka before going on to the party. Jennie had too much to drink too fast, and her boyfriend got angry at her for ruining the evening's plans. He took her car keys (a whisper of gratitude from me) and left her there alone.

Jennie had told her parents that she was going to spend the night with a girlfriend. "And now I can't get over to Cathy's because I can't drive my car, and my parents will find out that I didn't stay there, and they won't ever let me go out again. And so I called you, because you always, like, help me out, and I don't know what to do, and I'm scared to be here alone. Could you maybe come get me and take me to Cathy's house or something?"

"Well, have you tried calling Cathy? Maybe she or her parents could come get you?"

"Nnnoooo. . . . See, I can't ask her parents because they're not home either this weekend, only my parents don't know that. And I did call, but Cathy isn't home because I guess she's already at that party I was supposed to go to, and I don't know how to call her there. And, Dr. Mohrmann, *please* don't tell my parents."

They don't teach this stuff in medical school or in pediatric residencies.

Over the next hour or so, I arranged for the Daughertys' next-door neighbors to take her in for the night. The following afternoon, a contrite and terrified Jennie called to beg me not to tell her parents what had happened. I agreed to keep mum on one condition: no more drinking, period. If I had any reason to think she was drinking again, I would tell her parents immediately—no second chance. "Oh, thank you, Dr. Mohrmann. No, I've really learned my lesson. No more alcohol for me."

A few months later, I got a call at work from the guidance counselor at a local high school. A couple of Jennie's friends, concerned about her drinking in school, had come to the counselor with their worries. She confronted Jennie, who tearfully admitted to it and pleaded with the counselor to call me instead of her parents. The counselor agreed only to call me first. Jennie then left for home—school was out for the day—and the counselor called me as she had promised, but intended next to tell Mr. and Mrs. Daugherty. I convinced her, without much difficulty, to let me be the one to tell the Daughertys and talk with them about options for what to do next. As soon as I hung up, I called Jennie's parents and found them both at home. Jennie had not yet arrived, but they expected her any minute. I asked if I could come over to talk with them about something to do with Jennie and said I would like for her to be present for the conversation too. They were polite—or fearful—enough not to push for information over the phone, so I left them wondering what news awaited them.

I walked slowly to my car, thankful that this was not my afternoon in the clinic, and spent the short drive to their house pondering how to talk about this and what to recommend. Jennie answered my knock on their door.

She hissed under her breath, "You promised me you wouldn't tell them."

"Only if you didn't do it again, Jennie. I'm sorry. I have to. This is too important."

She turned away with a resigned shrug and led me into the living room, where her parents sat waiting, wary half-smiles on their faces. I explained that I had come to talk with them about my concerns about Jennie's use of alcohol, and then I told them about the counselor's call. They were dismayed, but not shocked. Mrs. Daugherty told me that their neighbor had told them about the previous episode right after it happened. They had talked with Jennie about it then and had received, and chosen to believe, the same assurances Jennie had given me. They had had no further indication that she was drinking at all, much less at school.

All through our conversation, Jennie sat silent and morose, refusing every invitation to join in, defend herself, or participate in the decisions being made. We agreed, and told Jennie that we took her silence for consent, that she would see a substance abuse counselor as soon as possible and, depending on the counselor's advice, perhaps begin attending meetings of Alcoholics Anonymous. Her parents were clearly determined to see it through this time. I left the house believing we were doing the right things for Jennie's well-being but still felt rotten, as though I had betrayed her. Perhaps the betrayal had really happened with the first drinking episode I was aware of and my failure to pursue it with her. I had not taken it seriously enough—or, perhaps, had taken my promise of confidentiality too seriously?—to seek help for her, even knowing her personality as I did, her need for whatever could take her away from herself.

Fortunately, Jennie did well, at least as far as alcohol was concerned, after that. I have had word of her, off and on, since I moved away. She graduated from high school and was accepted into a program that would train her to be an employee of a large, international firm. It meant she had to move several hundred miles away for the yearlong training course and carried the prospect of her being assigned to positions equally far afield. She lasted a little over a month at the training center. Within a year of her return she married and has since had two children (so much for nonfunctioning ovaries). Last I heard, she and the children were living back at home with her parents.

Chapter 8

Power and Powerlessness

REYE SYNDROME is such an odd disease, enigmatic and terrible. During one year in the early 1980s, I cared for eight children with the disease; only two of them survived. Over the previous ten years or so, Reye syndrome had seemed to arise from nowhere and gradually increased in scope to become, not exactly common, but distressingly frequent in occurrence and devastating in effect. Children who had appeared to be recovering normally from a minor respiratory illness, influenza, or the ubiquitous and generally benign chicken pox developed a strange listlessness punctuated by bouts of protracted vomiting. If the disease progressed, as it usually did, these symptoms would be followed in short order by an agitated delirium, then coma, which, in too many cases, ended in death.

The physiologic derangements of the disease resulted in marked swelling of brain tissue, with a concomitant increase in intracranial pressure, the cause of the coma and subsequent death. Many organs—the liver is a good example—swell in the presence of damage done by infection, injury, or intoxication, but, although the disorder itself may damage the organ, the swelling usually does not. Of the body's organs, only the brain is encased in bone. Once the skull's joints are sealed, by the end of the first two to three years of life, the cranium forms an unyielding wall against which the swelling brain can only batter and bruise itself. Therefore swelling alone, regardless of its cause, can destroy a brain in part or in whole. The increase in pressure within the skull cannot burst the bones; it can only compress and kill the brain tissue—and as the brain goes, so goes the person.

The most frightful thing about Reye syndrome was how quickly and dramatically it caused the brain to balloon with excess fluid. The only avenues available for treating the swollen brain of a child with Reye syndrome were measures designed to decrease intracranial pressure—crude, ham-handed interventions; there is no fine-tuning yet available—until the disease exhausted itself and the danger was past. The typical course of a patient with Reye syndrome was but a few days from the first signs of trouble to either death or recovery. Thus, the disease was an intense crisis for patient, family, and medical staff.

After the year in which I had eight patients with Reye syndrome, and also attended two national conferences seeking to understand the cause and improve the treatment of the disease, the number of children afflicted began to drop dramatically. Two years later I had no patients with Reye syndrome. It is now virtually extinct, and it is little clearer why it disappeared than why it emerged in the first place.

I sometimes think about the parents of the children who died around 1980 from this disease. I wonder what it is like to try to tell the story of such a shattering event in one's life to listeners who are likely never to have heard of the disease that killed your child. What might that kernel of unintelligibility do to the putative healing power of "telling one's story"? That is, how much does it matter to a narrative encounter that the listener be able to grasp the account within known categories of catastrophe, such as cancer, meningitis, or an automobile accident? Would the strangeness of the diagnosis of Reye syndrome be likely to intensify or to dampen the listener's ability to respond empathically to the bereaved storyteller? I picture parents recounting their child's fatal course only to be met with curiosity—"What's Reye syndrome?"—instead of attention to their profound loss. I wonder if some parents have been tempted to rewrite the story, substituting a more recognizable diagnosis—meningitis might work, with its neurological symptoms and often similar time course—in order to circumvent the obstacle of unfamiliarity and get directly to the central matter of loss.

Beyond matters of narrative integrity, I also wonder whether the parents of a child who died because of a disease that appeared and disappeared within such a short span of time—less than ten years for its epidemic phase—might be even more likely than parents of children with more customary disorders to ask the difficult "why" questions. For a child born a few years earlier or later, there was no Reye syndrome lying in ambush. Even knottier than the puzzle of why a child develops cancer or meningitis or is killed by a drunk driver—events that strike a predictable number of children each year—is the question of why a child is cut down by an affliction that seems to have had no or few victims before or after that discrete outbreak. At least for me, and so I assume also for some parents touched more closely than I by the disease, the short and terrible history of Reye syndrome evokes queries about the roles of randomness and order in our world, questions that ultimately reach back to basic cosmological or theological understandings of transcendent involvement, or its absence, in our lives—as "why" questions about life-and-death matters always do.

But on that autumn Saturday in 1981, Carey's parents were not asking those sorts of "why" questions—not yet, at any rate. They were too stunned, nodding slowly as I explained the next steps in their child's treatment and eased them into the news of possible outcomes. Carey, their ten-year-old daughter, had been out of school a couple of days with a flu-like illness, not too bad at first, but bad enough to keep this active child in bed. On Friday she seemed more mopey than usual and vomited quite a few times, but they attributed that to the ongoing effects of the illness and to a moodiness not unheard of in children her age. By Saturday morning she had stopped vomiting but was really quite droopy, so they called her doctor. After examining her, he was concerned that the viral infection was now causing encephalitis, which would explain her lethargy, and referred her to us at the medical center.

The resident called me late Saturday morning to tell me about her. He reported that, far from being lethargic, Carey was quite combative, talking nonsense and flailing about when they tried to do anything with her. The ambulance attendants said that this behavior had started during the hour's ride to the hospital. Given the many cases I had seen over the past couple of years, my mind immediately registered "stage two Reye syndrome," and my heart sank even as my brain shifted into formulating what needed to be done. I talked with the resident about what I thought and the lab tests needed to make the diagnosis certain, and I prepared to come to the hospital.

I was at Carey's bedside twenty minutes later, and I listened to the history of her illness from her father as I examined her. She was a stocky white child who was above average in height; were it not for her delirium—her long, fair hair whipped back and forth as she thrashed around—I would have said she looked quite healthy. All the information from Carey's history and the physical examination confirmed my initial assumption, as did the lab results when they returned: Reye syndrome, stage two. Carey's mother arrived just then; she had picked up their son, Carey's older brother, from a nearby college while her husband rode with Carey in the ambulance. I sat down with the family to explain, as well as I could, this baffling disease and its seemingly arbitrary course. I was heartened by the fact that she had spent a long time, as much as twenty-four hours, in the first stage of apathy and vomiting. Slow progression through the stages often heralded a good outcome, that is, a disease course that would not go beyond the second stage of agitated delirium. But I had also seen and read of too many children whose course did not fit this norm to rely on such predictors.

I told her parents and brother what we were watching for, what we were doing now, and what we would do if she moved into the next stage. Their reactions were what I had learned to expect with such news: tears, hands clutching for each other, bewilderment, and insistence that I do whatever I knew to do to make her better. There was no questioning, no call for a second opinion, only a deep and desperate trust; and although I probably appeared competent and, I believe, was being both kind and forthcoming with them, there really had not been reason yet for them to trust me so wholeheartedly.

I think such initial, intense reliance has to do with two intersecting characteristics of situations like this one. First is the obvious seriousness of the child's illness and her parents' manifest helplessness in the face of it: they must trust someone. Second, her parents include me within their general confidence in the medical profession, the institution of hospitals, and this medical center in particular. At a not-quite-conscious level, I expect they believe that their state's medical school hospital would not let me be there, calling the shots affecting the life of their daughter, if I were not entirely reliable. This sort of unquestioning confidence in the physician seems to be the rule (with, of course, its inevitable exceptions) for patients and families in the midst of medical crises. Parents almost always gave their children into my keeping gratefully, without asking what my board scores were, whether I had had adequate C.M.E. (Continuing Medical Education) credits that year, or whether there had been malpractice charges brought against me. In Carey's case, I think her parents heard only that I could identify this unimaginable affliction; that I had seen it many times; that I could make sense of it, such as it was; and that I knew what to do next—even while I was telling them that the "what to do" might not make a bit of difference, but that it was indeed what one did.

Over the next couple of hours, as her family watched by her bedside, Carey subsided into the coma of stage three Reye syndrome. At first they were pleased that she was so much less combative and that she seemed to be sleeping easily. Unfortunately, I had to disillusion them. What they were seeing was her transition between stages. The periods of "sleep" were lapses into coma, from which she was able to be roused less and less often. She had to be moved to the intensive care unit (the pediatric unit was full, so it would have to be the adult I.C.U.), where we would put in an intracranial pressure (I.C.P.) monitor. They greeted the news stoically: I had explained it earlier, and they had expected it, sort of.

While I arranged her transfer to the I.C.U., the resident paged the neurosurgeon who would have to place the "bolt," or the I.C.P. monitor. This device is a catheter inserted through a hole drilled into the skull. It traverses the tissue of the brain's cortex to reach the ventricles, which lie deep inside the cranium, matched reservoirs full of the cerebrospinal fluid (C.S.F.), which bathes the entire brain and spinal column. There the tip of the catheter rests, gauging the pressure within the C.S.F. system, and thus the I.C.P., by measuring pressure transmitted to the fluid within the catheter. An elegant setup, if you forget the part about the catheter tracking through the cerebrum to get there. In swollen brains, the ventricles can be hard to find, squashed almost flat by the expanding cerebral hemispheres. The neurosurgeon may have to make several attempts—all blind or, perhaps I should say, guided only by the internal vision of knowledge and experience—several passes through the brain, taking neurons with him as he probes. This is not like putting a catheter into a bladder or an arm vein. Neurosurgeons assure me that because we all have so much more brain tissue than we need—or, rather, than we use—even multiple passes with the bolt are no problem; they do not see untoward consequences of this procedure. Nevertheless, I wonder if anyone can distinguish, with any certainty, the results of bolt placement from the effects of the disease that required pressure monitoring in the first place. Each time I watched a neurosurgeon move the catheter in and out, up and down, searching for the ventricle, I envisioned a little bulldozer taking out pieces of the landscape with each pass: there goes the dog's name, there the first song I learned in kindergarten, there my newfound skill at pedaling a two-wheeler.

Fortunately, Carey was apparently early into stage three; I even wondered at first if I had jumped the gun in calling for the bolt to be placed. There was no problem finding her ventricles, just a smooth, one-shot pass and an initial pressure reading well within the normal range. Maybe overzealous management, but at least we knew her I.C.P. was all right for now, and we had a way to check it and therefore did not have to rely solely on nonspecific signs. I was relieved to have her in the I.C.U. and so intimately monitored that I could set aside some of my chronic anxiety about assessment skills, an unease that comes with the territory. By then I had already learned the important lesson that appropriate confidence in one's abilities is ultimately built upon that kind of concern. The absence of uncertainty—the too-quick belief that you have it right—is the foundation not of competence but of carelessness. I made sure the residents were clear on what to watch for and do, checked in with her parents, and went home to change for dinner at the home of friends.

I made it to the dinner party but had been there less than an hour when I was paged. Carey's intracranial pressure had suddenly gone up, and the residents were instituting the necessary measures to get it back under control. But it was clear that they were worried and unsure of themselves—this was not an everyday task, by any means—so I said my farewells and returned to the hospital. Truth to tell, I was glad to do so. My concern for Carey and where the disease might take her that evening made it impossible for me to relax with my friends. I was better off being at the hospital, whether or not my being there made any difference to Carey's well-being. Slowly, over the next few hours, our interventions got her I.C.P. to level off at a point only slightly above normal, although we were not sanguine about how long that stability would last.

At about two o'clock on Sunday morning, I received a page in the I.C.U., where we were tinkering with Carey's medications and ventilator settings to bring her I.C.P. back down after it had strayed upward once again. Strange, I thought, everyone who might page me is here with me. The pager turned out to be a local pediatrician, working in the emergency room of the private hospital a few blocks away. He professed delight at finding me in the hospital because he was seeing an eight-year-old boy about whom he was, he admitted, a little worried and whom he wanted to send over to me for a second opinion. He said that the child seemed to have only an ordinary viral illness of short duration and did not look too sick, but his blood pressure was surprisingly low; he thought he might need our attention.

"Sure," I said, thinking he probably just needed a lot of intravenous fluids. "Send him on."

Seeing that Carey's I.C.P. was back under control, I went down with the senior resident to meet this new patient, David, in the hospital's first-floor triage center. He looked dreadful. His blood pressure was so low as to be almost unmeasurable, but he was awake and panicky, his gray face and lips calling for his mother, for help. David was in profound shock, for no discernible reason. We immediately began filling his circulatory system with fluid, with antibiotics, with steroids, with drugs to boost his blood pressure—to no avail. Nothing changed. His pressure remained too low for life. His panic subsided as his energy waned. All through the remainder of that night we labored over his little body, perplexed at the cause of this disaster, exhausting all our means of fending it off. I called colleagues for suggestions, but they were as puzzled as I by his lack of response to our treatments and at a loss to say what else we could possibly do for him.

Around five o'clock that morning, at a point in the battle for David's life when we could only wait to see if our treatment measures would have any effect, having no remaining options, I left him in the care of the senior resident and went to check on Carey—whose condition was, fortunately, remaining stable—and to lie down for a short nap. Carey's parents later told me that they came to visit their daughter and saw me dozing on the sofa in the nurse's lounge beside the I.C.U. They said, "We saw you there, and we knew everything would be all right as long as you were around."

They could not know how hard that was for me to hear. They were attributing extraordinary healing power to me, such that my mere presence ensured a good outcome for their daughter. But they had no idea of my powerlessness. No idea that, at the same time they were rejoicing in my being there, another child was slipping away, and I could not stop him going.

David died later that morning. His blood pressure never came up; his heart finally quit trying. Because of religious convictions, his mother would not consent to autopsy. David's blood and tissue cultures never grew any microorganism we could blame for his death. A year or so later, I began reading reports of a newly recognized toxic shock syndrome, characterized by rapid onset of shock, severe and refractory low blood pressure, and often a quick progression to death. Was that what David had? I do not know. I talked with his mother a month or so after his death, to go over what had happened that night, and I had to admit to her that I still did not know what had killed her son, or why—nor what I should or could have done differently for him.

Carey did remarkably well. By late Sunday afternoon, her intracranial pressure needed no further manipulation to keep it from rising and then gradually began to slip back into the normal range. In the parlance of Reye syndrome, she did not progress beyond stage three. Forty-eight hours later, we were ready to remove the I.C.P. monitor. Before doing that, however, we withdrew, one by one, all the measures in place to keep her I.C.P. down while we could still gauge the effect on her pressure. By Wednesday morning, all that was left to be done was to take her off ventilatory support. Respiratory control—specifically hyperventilation, that is, rapid deep breathing to keep carbon dioxide levels low—is a fundamental technique for managing intracranial pressure. Carey had been sedated and intubated, with the tracheal tube then connected to a ventilator, at the same time her bolt had been placed. Now it was time to remove the tube from her trachea, but there was a problem.

A routine blood gas determination showed, oddly, that her oxygen level was low. There was nothing about Reye syndrome that should cause that. I listened to her lungs and heard crackles in both bases. Pneumonia? Why? Because of that "flu" she had had? An X ray of her chest provided the answer. At some point, perhaps at the time she was intubated, Carey had inhaled stomach contents. That is, acidic fluid from her stomach had rolled up into her esophagus and spilled down her airways deep into her lung tissue. It apparently had taken this long for the inflammation induced by the aspirated gastric juices to worsen to the point of interfering with oxygen exchange. This was a potentially disastrous complication; if the damage was widespread enough, Carey's lungs could become unventilatable. She was certainly not going to be extubated. Because her I.C.P. had been normal for more than a day, we took out the bolt but kept her on the ventilator and started antibiotics against the possibility that her inflamed lungs had also become infected.

We had lightened Carey's sedation to enable her to breathe fully on her own when we extubated her, so she was awake and aware of what was going on. I was pleased to see her alertness—a good sign that the Reye syndrome had not left behind major brain damage—but it also meant having to explain to her why the tube was going to stay in and that we would have to continue breathing for her in order to put oxygen in at pressures that would allow her blood to be adequately nourished. She took it well, probably aided by her being still dazed, and just nodded her understanding. Then I went to talk with her family.

Carey's parents and her brother had established themselves in the one big waiting room, a few floors down from the I.C.U., that served virtually all the critical care areas and operating rooms in this 1950s-era hospital. The room—really more a large space off the main hallway, without doors—was like an indoor tent city, strewn with blankets, pillows, plastic bags packed with toiletries and a change of underwear, fast food cartons, and countless paper coffee cups. Each waiting family claimed a certain area of the room, circled the chairs, and camped out. Once each day, housekeeping staff or volunteer aides came by to insist that the chairs be lined up again in their former fashion; as soon as they departed, the camps were rebuilt. This was the only place available for waiting out a lingering crisis, except for one small side room, off the main space, which was usually reserved for the most recently bereaved family, there being told the bad news and allowed to grieve privately. Most often the little room stood empty; no one wanted to claim it, much less be invited into it by a doctor.

News of anything short of death was usually conveyed out in the open, in the midst of this expanded waiting family. What privacy there was could be obtained only by the circled chairs and a soft voice: not a brilliant setup. Carey's family had claimed a segment of the room nearest the hallway, an area that everyone had to walk through to get to other parts of the room but with the best vantage point for seeing who was getting off the elevator. I had become aware in the past few days that the expression on my face as I stepped off the elevator and headed in their direction had the effect of elating or depressing them long before I was in earshot. Why should they think—how could they believe it?—that my facial expression was more likely to have been influenced by my elevator companions than by their daughter's condition? After the first misreading—I looked so glum, but the news was so good—I realized I had to pay attention to this. It had been difficult to convince them of the goodness of the news when they were still feeling the effects of the adrenalin surge I had triggered by my distant, lowering visage. (Who knows whom or what I had been pulling away from to look so grim?) This was an aspect of my "power" I had not considered before: not just my words but my demeanor determined their emotional state for the few days during which they understood their daughter's life to be in my hands. They scanned my every posture, gesture, and tone for clues to their future. I was not so much an oracle as a deck of tarot cards, dealing them their fate with each move.

This day I came over to them with my face arranged in what I hoped (should I practice this in front of a mirror?) was an honest combination of bad news and guarded optimism, whatever that looks like. At any rate, something showed because they greeted me warily. Our last conversation, earlier that morning, had been all sunny: I.C.P. is great; we're going up to get her off everything; I'll come back and report when we've got it done; you're on the way home now. Great joy, gratitude, relief—we've really all survived this. The rest of the waiting room rejoiced with them. I basked in the warmth of their pleasure. But now I was back with something different to say. "There's been a complication we need to talk about."

Carey's brother sat cross-legged on the floor. His parents were in chairs drawn close on either side of him, forming a three-sided box. I sat on the floor at the open end to close the square and draw us into a more private space. I expected others in the room, waiting for news of their loved ones, to respect it; it is what they wanted for themselves.

I explained what was going on, about the aspiration pneumonia and what we now had to do to get her through it. I was quite sure the Reye syndrome was done with now; it would not revive and strike again. But the pneumonia was no mere diversion. It was serious, and we would have to see how Carey did over the next day or so before we could say with any certainty that she was out of danger. They gulped and took it all in, shocked by the reversal, unprepared to face another life-threatening problem.

Carey's brother said firmly, "She beat the Reye syndrome. She can beat this too." They all smiled bravely, asked the right questions, nodded at the answers, and thanked me for coming to talk with them. As I waited for the elevator, I looked back and saw them holding each other, crying.

For the next two days, Carey needed increasing amounts of oxygen and higher ventilator pressures to get sufficient oxygen into her bloodstream. And then, on Friday, she began slowly to improve as her young, healthy body's healing mechanisms gradually repaired the sacs and airways of her damaged lungs. After two more days, she was able to come off the ventilator. On Monday, Carey left the I.C.U., with great rejoicing and hugs all around. (She had been warmly adopted by the nurses in the adult I.C.U., so glad, they said, to care for a young person who got well!) By Wednesday afternoon, less than two weeks from the start of her adventure, she was home.

A few weeks later, Carey and her parents came for a follow-up visit. She had a completely normal examination, with no signs of residual damage to her brain or her lungs. They brought me a beautiful, big rubber plant, which lived in my house for many years, until it could finally no longer resist the toxic effects of my brown thumb—and Carey shyly handed me one of her school pictures from fifth grade, on the back of which she had pledged her undying love for me. I look at it now and wonder how she is—she is in her thirties now—and I am so grateful for the wonderful resilience of childhood.

I cannot remember Carey, however, without also remembering David. The contrast between the two situations—one in which the family saw me as so potent a shield against the disease threatening their daughter, the other in which my impotence was plain—brought me up short at the time, and it still does. Together Carey and David showed me, that long and difficult night twenty-plus years ago, not only the contingency and limitations of the healer's "power"—about which I had already learned quite a bit—but also the fact that such power as doctors have is in large part ascribed to us gratuitously by the patients and families who require us to accept and use their often burdensome gift wisely and with compassion.

Chapter 9

Letting Go and Going On

BECAUSE I WAS THE director of the P.I.C.U., I got the call from the pediatric surgeon, who wanted a bed for a new patient. It was November 1982. There was a baby girl about 100 miles upstate who was thought to have pyloric stenosis—a tight stricture at the junction of the stomach and small intestine—and needed to be transferred to our medical center for surgical correction of the problem. Although she was only a few days old, she could not be admitted to the N.I.C.U. because she had been at home briefly, and the N.I.C.U. did not allow "outside" babies, exposed to nonhospital germs, to enter. But she definitely needed intensive care, the surgeon told me, not just the regular infant ward. Her vomiting, the characteristic symptom of pyloric stenosis, had made her quite sick. Her blood urea nitrogen was high, suggesting a significant degree of dehydration.

I briefly quizzed the surgeon about the diagnosis: most babies with pyloric stenosis are male and few become so sick this early in life. He agreed this would be an unusual example of the disorder, but nevertheless that was how it had been presented to him. There was no question that she needed to be in the P.I.C.U. I arranged for the bed and awaited her arrival, wondering if she would turn out to be my patient instead of his. I was not convinced she had a surgical problem. There are other causes for high blood urea nitrogen levels and vomiting in a newborn, most of them originating in the kidneys.

At that time, in addition to directing the P.I.C.U., I was acting as the nephrologist, the kidney specialist, on our pediatric faculty. Our "real" pediatric nephrologist had moved away more than a year before, and the department chairman had asked me to take charge of the renal patients until a replacement could be found. At that point in my career, I agreed to almost anything I was asked to do. I still had the "chief resident complex," not unusual among academic clinicians, that admits to no limitations of ability, time, or energy. It could have been a disastrous decision on my part, but that is not the way it turned out, fortunately, for I filled the "acting" position for four years. I enjoyed refreshing and expanding my knowledge of the disordered physiology involved in childhood kidney disease, and the patients and their families were a pleasure to work with. I had reliable and knowledgeable support from both the nephrologists on the adult medicine faculty and, by telephone, a group of pediatric nephrologists at a university medical center a few hundred miles away. With their guidance, I reorganized the renal clinic into a smoothly running operation that was getting an increasing number of referrals from around the state and shifted most of our patients who needed dialysis from hemodialysis to peritoneal dialysis.[1]

So I was the nephrologist manqué, and my newly sprouted kidney antennae told me that the baby girl on her way to the P.I.C.U. might be more in my field than in that of the surgeons. The baby's name was Lindsey. (Months later, her parents, Vonnie and Tony Leaphart, told us that their intention had been to call her by her middle name, Erin. But because the doctors and nurses all called her by her first name—Lindsey— from the start, they also came to think of her that way and eventually, they said, came to prefer that name.) After Lindsey's arrival in the P.I.C.U., it took only a brief examination and an abdominal X ray, plus a careful history from her parents, to convince the surgeons that she did not have pyloric stenosis and to convince me that she did indeed have some kind of bad kidney problem.

Further investigation not only confirmed that conviction but also revealed that, because of her markedly abnormal kidneys, Lindsey would soon require dialysis and, ultimately, a kidney transplant. The biopsy, which was done several weeks later when she was more stable and somewhat stronger, showed that her kidneys were composed of multiple cysts and virtually no normal-appearing or potentially functional tissue. The malformed structure did not fit any previously described pattern; the pathologists sent slides from the biopsy to experts in infant kidneys all over the country, but no one could put a definitive name to Lindsey's kidney disorder. However, her parents and I knew its practical name: disaster. Dialyzing an infant is not an easy task, but it was the only option available if Lindsey was to grow big enough and strong enough to receive a kidney transplant, her only real hope of survival. We started peritoneal dialysis, with the placement of a catheter into her abdominal cavity; hemodialysis machines could not accommodate the tiny size of a baby's blood vessels.

The difficulties of achieving and maintaining balance in Lindsey's fluid and electrolyte levels, and of keeping her adequately nourished, meant that she had to stay in the P.I.C.U. for some time. During those weeks, Vonnie lived nearby and spent most of each day and evening with her, while Tony and their other daughter, Marci, made do at home and came to visit on the weekends. Anxious and tearful at times, at other times strong and determined that Lindsey would come through this, Vonnie forged a strong bond with the P.I.C.U. nursing staff and with me. In fact, she became almost like one of the staff, to the point that we sometimes caught ourselves falling into habits of joking that we did not usually display in front of parents. She took it all in good humor, glad, I think, to be part of the only world her baby daughter knew.

By the first of the year, it became clear that Lindsey needed more than we could offer her. She needed doctors with more expertise and experience in pediatric nephrology. Since she was now stable enough to travel, we transferred her to the medical center, in a nearby state, whose pediatric kidney specialists had been acting as my advisers. She stayed there for about three weeks, during which they performed the kidney biopsy and stabilized her dialysis regimen so that she no longer required intensive care. Then they sent her back to us to grow, as we all hoped, aiming for the critical weight at which she could become a realistic candidate for a transplant. We knew the odds were not in her favor.

For more than two months after that, Lindsey and Vonnie lived in a room on the ward where children with renal and metabolic disorders were cared for. Not only was Vonnie a constant and faithful attendant for Lindsey's needs but she also took under her wing other children on the ward who were there for long stretches of time, or in and out with some frequency, without family members of their own in attendance. Vonnie doted on them all, but Lindsey was her heart, and her heart was breaking. Tony was as deeply involved but could be there only one or two evenings a week. On weekends, and sometimes during the week, four-year-old Marci accompanied him to see her mother and baby sister. I still have a photo of Marci holding Lindsey; she is surrounded and held by her parents, and there is a proud big-sister smile on her face.

Lindsey would gain a little, lose a little. She would have a few good days of being alert, looking more like a three-month-old baby, almost ready to hold her head up, but then there would be several days of listlessness and more trouble feeding. She never became very interested in food, and she continued to vomit with regularity, even with blood chemistries more nearly normal. By March, we could no longer fool ourselves into believing that she was going to be able to grow to the point of being a candidate for kidney transplant. She had started having recurrent infections, including one bout of peritonitis that, fortunately, could be handled without removing the dialysis catheter.

A week or two before Easter, Lindsey's parents and I had a long conversation about the reality of the situation. I had talked with my consultants at the other medical center, who now knew Lindsey almost as well as I did, and they had agreed that there were no options left to us. I discussed this with the Leapharts: that Lindsey was not going to be able to receive a transplant, that the peritoneal dialysis—which was becoming increasingly inefficient, her blood chemistries ever more difficult to control—was not going to work much longer, and that hemodialysis was not possible. Lindsey was outrunning what we could do for her. They knew it; they had probably known it before I did. After tears and painful silences, they asked what we were to do now. "We just don't want her to suffer, Dr. Mohrmann. What's it going to be like for her?"

I told them that we could take one of two paths. We could stop the dialysis, take out her peritoneal catheter, and keep her hydrated and comfortable. They could hold her and love her until she died a quiet death, probably within a few days. She was likely to die without pain or struggle, either with an overwhelming infection or, more likely, as the result of rising levels of unfiltered chemicals in her blood. The alternative was to continue what we were doing, knowing it to be increasingly ineffective, but do no more than that and let death come when it would, by infection or chemical derangement. They could not accept stopping the dialysis, abandoning the only flicker of hope, the only possible—no matter how improbable—avenue of treatment and survival. We agreed to change nothing but to recognize that we were now heading for the end, without knowing how long that path might be. They planned to explain it to Marci in some fashion, to prepare her for Lindsey's coming death.

A few days later, I noted that Lindsey had developed symptoms of a respiratory infection, as she had a few times in the past. I told her parents and went to order the antibiotic I had used before, hoping to keep a viral cold from turning into a bacterial pneumonia, always a risk in someone in such a weakened condition. After a few minutes, Tony came to find me. He and Vonnie had talked after I left.

"If we're really not doing anything, Dr. Mohrmann, if we're really just waiting for her to die, why treat this? I thought we weren't going to do anything new, add anything to what we're doing. Do we have to do this?"

I sat back in the chair, humbled by their insight and my lack of it, my readiness to fall back on comfortable routines. "No, we don't have to. You're right. This is just the kind of thing we said we wouldn't do. I'm okay not treating this if you're sure it's okay with you."

"Absolutely, Dr. Mohrmann. Let's leave her alone."

The cold did not turn into pneumonia, but she lived for only another week, gradually losing strength and alertness. On the afternoon of Easter Sunday 1983, I was out in my yard, weeding and edging one of the flower beds, when my pager sounded, summoning me to call Lindsey's ward. The nurse who answered told me Lindsey had just died. I cleaned up and drove to the hospital. Vonnie, Tony, and Marci were there, had been there when she died. They were tearful, but not distraught. On the contrary, they were in awe, they told me, that Lindsey's anticipated death had finally come on a day when they were all there with her, when Marci was able to tell her goodbye, when they were dressed for a special occasion—in fact, on Easter Sunday.

In the months that followed, Vonnie and Tony came to my office several times to talk about what they had experienced and how they and Marci were doing. On one visit, they brought two large rocking chairs, one for the P.I.C.U. and one for me, each with a plaque on the back of the seat claiming the chair as Lindsey's memorial. I was very touched. The chair lived in my office until I left that job and since then has had a treasured place in my house—treasured not only because of its association with Lindsey and her family but also because it is my favorite reading chair, the chair that never fails to ease my aching back, which has lifted a few too many children onto examining tables over the years. The chair is, for me, a tangible reminder of the deep reciprocity that exists between doctor and patient, in which the harms and the healing flow in both directions. It is where I am sitting now as I write this story on my laptop.

Several months after Lindsey's death, her parents began talking very tentatively and fearfully about having another baby. They very much wanted another child. Lindsey had been carefully planned for and eagerly awaited. But they—especially Vonnie—were also quite concerned about the risk of having another child with Lindsey's kidney disease. I had talked with our pediatric geneticist, using what information I had from the pathologists and consulting nephrologists, about what that risk might be, but without a definite diagnosis with a known pattern of inheritance, it was not possible to give clear odds on the chance of the malformation recurring. The best we could offer was the not very helpful generalization that, in such situations, the risk of recurrence is usually 5 percent or less. At least that gave me something to add to the deliberations, whatever a one-in-twenty chance might mean when it is a prospect of reliving the heartbreaking and exhausting five months of Lindsey's life.

We discussed the question over and over. I emphasized how unlikely it was that another baby of theirs would have the same problem while admitting that, were it to recur, we would be able to do no more for the new baby than we had for Lindsey. Even being prepared to look for kidney disease immediately after birth, or, for that matter, before birth, would not make a significant difference in the outcome. Ultimately, the decision would have to come down to their willingness to take the risk, to balance it against their strong desire for another child, perhaps to focus on the 95 percent chance that the malformation would not recur. Tony was ready; Vonnie not quite. And so it went through a few visits. We discussed whether, were she to become pregnant, they should plan on delivering in our medical center, whether, if they stayed in their hometown, they should keep the same pediatrician—which gave me the opportunity to remind them that their pediatrician had done precisely the right thing by sending Lindsey to us and could not have been expected also to have made an accurate diagnosis of such an unusual abnormality.

Finally, they decided to "try again," and Vonnie soon became pregnant. The pregnancy was full of worry but otherwise uncomplicated. Prenatal ultrasounds detected no abnormalities in the developing fetus. Their baby girl was entirely healthy with demonstrably normal kidneys. Much to my surprise and delight, Vonnie and Tony named her for me. They call her Maggie. Alongside my picture of Marci holding Lindsey, I have one of eight-year-old Marci and two-year-old Maggie, in their spring finery, Easter 1987.

Chapter 10

Suspending Disbelief

DURING MY CAREER, accompanying children and their parents through the travails of illness and suffering as their attending physician has been important for their care, I believe, and certainly for my edification. But being part of their struggles, healings, or deaths has also often been a moving experience of beauty and grace. Beyond the lessons to be learned, the healing to be invoked, and the solace to be given by "being there," the inexpressible joy of being a doctor lies in the sheer privilege of recognizing moments of transcendence in an inexplicable healing, of witnessing the fathomless courage of some children and parents, of receiving a trusting child's handclasp.

⇘ Jack

TOWARD THE END of my stint as acting nephrologist, I got a request from a colleague, a neonatologist, for a consult. The baby he was concerned about, Jack Hogan, had been born two days before, after an uncomplicated labor and delivery at the end of a full-term, equally uncomplicated pregnancy. Jack had looked splendid at birth, well grown and strong, with no detectible abnormalities. His mother, in contrast, had become very ill immediately after giving birth with a clotting disorder known to be a complication of delivery.

Mrs. Hogan had delivered Jack at a community hospital an hour or so away and had been transferred to our medical intensive care unit as soon as the seriousness of her condition was recognized. The baby had been brought to our nursery at the same time, in case his mother became able to breastfeed. On initial examination, Jack had looked like any other healthy newborn. However, on his second day of life he was noted to be edematous, that is, puffy because of excess fluid in his tissues. Evaluation of the swelling had revealed very low levels of protein, particularly albumin, in his blood and a large amount of protein, but no blood, in his urine. Although these findings easily explained his edema, the cause of the protein loss in his urine was not so clear. Hence the call to me.

Jack looked like a normal, energetic newborn baby, with the exception of his definite puffiness. He had a downy mass of black hair on his well-shaped head, glowing brown skin, arms and legs going in all directions in response to my touch. The soft swelling encircled his eyes and fattened his cheeks, tracked along his spine, and ballooned his hands and feet. My investigation of the relevant textbooks suggested only congenital nephrotic syndrome, a very unusual disorder affecting newborns with just such signs as Jack manifested, but I was reluctant to saddle him with that diagnosis, not only because of my inexperience but also because of its grim prognosis. Infants born with nephrotic syndrome—a disease very different from the sort of nephrotic syndrome that appears in older chil dren—fare very poorly. There was no treatment available other than kidney transplant, but getting such children to grow to a size and state of health sufficient for successful transplantation was virtually impossible given the constant loss of protein, the most essential component of growth. Dialysis would not help because the problem was not a kidney that could not filter toxins from the blood; the filtration function worked normally. It was the protein leak that mattered, and dialysis could not fix that. Most children with congenital nephrotic syndrome, after months of chronic malnutrition and recurrent infections, died before their first birthday, usually as a result of a final, overwhelming infection against which they had little defense, so many vital germ-fighting proteins having been lost through their disordered kidneys.

I presented Jack's situation to my supporting nephrologists at the distant medical center, who had helped me through so many difficult cases. They too believed he had congenital nephrosis and suggested some additional tests, all of which confirmed that diagnosis by eliminating other, more remote possibilities. We knew he would need a renal biopsy to make the diagnosis definite and agreed that when he was a bit older and stronger he would come to their center to have that procedure done. We rehearsed the aspects of his care—nutrition, protection from infection, close follow-up—that would be necessary to help him get to that older, stronger point.

Jack's mother was still in the adult I.C.U., heavily sedated, his father in vigil at his wife's bedside. I decided that Mr. Hogan did not need yet another strange face coming with more difficult news for him to shoulder, so I communicated with him through the neonatologist. Jack would be all right for the near future. He was eating well, maintaining his blood protein at its low level, and not yet suffering any ill effects of the protein loss, other than the edema. If this was indeed congenital nephrotic syndrome, his parents would have time to get used to the idea as they watched Jack first fail to thrive and then dwindle away over the next year—at least, that was the picture I had formed based on my books and my consultations with colleagues.

I continued to look in on Jack, who remained much the same. A few days later I heard that Mrs. Hogan was recovering from her critical illness and was out of the I.C.U., a minor miracle in itself given the severity of her illness. Mother and baby went home the next week, with an appointment to see me in renal clinic in two weeks, when Jack would be almost a month old, at which time I would explain everything to them.

Both parents accompanied the baby to his first clinic visit. Mrs. Hogan, though still quite thin after her ordeal, looked as though she was rapidly regaining her strength. She was tall and graceful, with an expressive, open face and a soft voice. Jack's father was equally gentle of tone and demeanor, quietly solicitous of his recovering wife's needs. My first impression of them—it is as real to me now, writing this some twenty years later, as it was then, in that small examining room—was that they were an extraordinary couple, compellingly attractive not only in their physical beauty but in their manifest serenity and joy. They were simply radiant, giving off a warmth that seemed to embrace me and all the rest of the surrounding world in its glow. I was immediately at ease with them and, thus, all the more chagrined at the news I had to give. Jack had gained an appropriate amount of weight but still had about the same degree of edema as I had noted in the nursery, so I knew his protein levels would still be low. He had shown no signs of infection and continued to be an eager eater. They considered him a perfect baby. They were clearly in love with this child, their first, rejoicing simultaneously in his presence and in his mother's return to health.

As gently but as uncompromisingly as I could, I told them the probable explanation for Jack's edema. I drew out for them the causal connections between protein loss in the urine, low protein levels in the blood, failure to grow, and susceptibility to infection. I told them the survival statistics. They looked up at me from time to time as I spoke, then looked back at their son, asleep in his father's arms. When I finished, they were silent for a minute.

Jack's mother looked up at me, her eyes glinting with unshed tears, but with a broad smile on her face nevertheless. "Thank you for telling us, Dr. Mohrmann. You've been very clear. Thanks for telling us everything. But, you see, we know God will heal Jack."

Mr. Hogan beamed. "That's right. Just the way he healed you," he said, nodding toward his wife.

I was both flummoxed and charmed. Such intense certainty, such peace in their assurance—quite amazing. All I could say was something like "Well, I surely hope so." Then I pushed a bit to be sure their belief in a coming miracle did not mean they intended to disregard my recommendations or fail to keep clinic appointments.

"No, no," they said together, shaking their heads and looking serious. Mr. Hogan clarified: "This is how God works. Of course, we'll do everything you ask. That's how he'll be healed."

I made a brief stab at explaining to them that nothing I was recommending would do anything to heal Jack's kidneys, but would only—and at best—help protect him for a while from the effects of the disorder. But in the face of their patient serenity my protestations soon faltered and ceased. I drew blood from Jack for testing, obtained a sample of his urine, and arranged to see Jack again in a month. The lab results showed he was losing as much protein as before and that his serum albumin was no higher than it had been in the nursery.

I saw Jack monthly for the next several months. Each time he had grown appropriately and attained the next set of normal developmental milestones. At each visit, his edema was a little less, his serum albumin a little higher, his urine protein a little lower. Each month I called my colleagues in nephrology for a session of mutual telephonic head scratching. What was happening here? We did not know of anything that looked like what he had but could get better on its own. And yet it was. Each month, Jack's mother gently reminded me—in tones of pure joy—that *she* understood what was happening to her son.

When Jack was six months old, he sat up without support, babbled, and acted in every way like a happy, healthy six-month-old should. He was the normal weight and length for his age. There was no edema and no protein in his urine; his blood protein levels were normal. He was now the right age and size for a renal biopsy, but there was no longer a reason to do one.

"I don't understand it," I admitted, shaking my baffled head as Jack's mother and I stood together beside the examining table, enjoying his gurgling good health.

"I told you God would heal him," she said, with a light, teasing nudge of her elbow to my ribs. "See?" She did not try to suppress the grin, the laughter that bubbled up and blended with her son's excited giggles. I had to join them.

I called my consultants with this latest, confounding, wonderful news. "Well," one of the kidney specialists said, "obviously it wasn't congenital nephrotic syndrome. I don't know what it was, but it couldn't have been that if he got over it. Too bad we didn't get a biopsy earlier."

I saw Jack and his parents every six months until I moved away; he remained entirely healthy. After I left Charleston, Jack's mother called me every few years to say hello and to report on his progress. He is now a twenty-two-year-old college graduate, employed and married, with no hint of kidney disease. His mother is convinced that I was an entirely effective agent of Jack's healing. I do not believe I did anything that could count as a healing act. Yet, there is Jack, healed—of something.

What was wrong with Jack? I don't know for sure. I only know it isn't there anymore. Jack's parents have no question about what happened; they are certain that God healed their son of his incurable disorder. So, too, when Jennie Daugherty recovered fully from her almost-fatal lung disease, despite all prognostic evidence to the contrary, her parents were sure that their reliance on prayer had been vindicated. But their explanations of these wonderful occurrences leave other questions unanswered, questions that I am unable to dismiss. What about all the other children I have cared for, those who were also vigorously prayed over but were not healed and did not recover? Why would God pluck Mickey for some heavenly garden, as the troubling prayer cards at her wake claimed, but leave Jack and Jennie behind?

My nephrology colleagues handled the dilemma of Jack's healing with practiced ease. They had insisted from the start that his disorder could be nothing but congenital nephrotic syndrome. When he recovered fully, they said it could not have been that disease, ipso facto. The scientific training of physicians, as creative and far-seeing as it may enable us to be, also limits our ability to consider seriously events or findings that seem beyond the grasp of science. It becomes far more comfortable to assume that whatever is not now explainable by science either will be eventually or, should it prove incorrigibly inexplicable, is an illusion. Case closed.

But this case is not closed for me. In the name of all the unhealed children and of my belief in the profound goodness of God, I resist facile attributions of arbitrary divine intervention. In the face of what I have seen and know to have happened, I resist science's unsatisfactory "explanations" or outright dismissal of the perplexing marvels that, with remarkable frequency, confront medical professionals. I prefer to leave the questions unanswered, the cases open, and allow them to stay at the forefront of my experience, expanding my vision and deepening my capacity for wonder.

One Christmas Day I came to the hospital late in the morning to make my rounds. I was just beginning to read my patients' charts when I was called by a nurse on the "specialty ward," the area that housed mostly patients with cancer and heart disease. She had seen me arrive and knew I was the only pediatric attending in the hospital. One of her patients had just died, and she asked if I would mind coming to his room to pronounce the child dead and talk a little with his mother.

A few minutes later, I walked into the room and saw a boy of about four or five, bald and clad in Superman pajamas, lying on his side in a bed covered with and surrounded by a chaos of toys and crumpled Christmas wrapping paper. A woman, his mother, sat quietly on the end of his bed, looking down. I introduced myself to her, expressed my condolences, then leaned over the child and listened for a heartbeat to assure myself that he was indeed dead. I asked his mother and the nurse to tell me something of what had happened that morning. The story, which they told me together, corroborating and filling in for each other, was this:

Damian had had leukemia for two years. When he was admitted in relapse, a month or so earlier, his doctors were pessimistic about the possibility of achieving another remission. As the month progressed, it became clear that he would not survive this bout—in fact, his death was expected at any time—and all agreed that no "heroic" measures would be undertaken when he died. His mother, who understood and seemed to accept the inevitability of his death, had told the nurses several times that her one remaining hope was that he survive until Christmas. She had already purchased his gifts, all the things he had asked for, and wanted so much to have one more Christmas morning with him, to watch his pleasure in opening the gifts.

On Christmas morning she arrived early, huge sacks of presents in hand. Damian sat up in bed, opened and exclaimed over every gift, a process that took a few hours, there being so many. When the unwrapping was done, the nurse took his vital signs and had him stand up on the scale to be weighed. Damian then said he wanted to take a nap, so he lay down, leaving the joyful detritus of the morning scattered around him, pulled the covers to his chest, and went to sleep. And died.

How does one explain a four-year-old's exquisite timing? What makes it possible for a child to give such a gift to his mother, to delay his death—is that even the right phrase?—in order to give her a last Christmas morning with him? Damian was not healed, not obviously at any rate, but his story is as mysterious, as wonderful as Jack's or Jennie's.

Damian's Christmas morning death could be set aside as a simple coincidence, but, beginning with Sherry's death at the time of her anointing when I was an intern, I had become wary of using that label to explain away the baffling, even astounding events I was privileged to witness. During my residency and, even more so, during my years directing the P.I.C.U., I became aware of a remarkable phenomenon that ultimately put an end to any lingering reliance I might have had on coincidence as an explanatory escape. More times than I can count, I took care of or observed the care of children who were dying—clearly, hopelessly, inexorably—but would not die. For no fathomable reason, they hung on when every physiological measure, every scientific assay was "incompatible with life" and signaled that they should already be dead. Almost invariably, a child who would not die was accompanied by parents who would not accept the inevitable death, who continued to ask for any intervention possible despite manifest futility. Then, when the child's parents finally became resigned, ceased the useless fight, and began to mourn, I could return to the P.I.C.U. from my conversation with them and tell the nurses that the child would likely die within the next twenty-four hours. I was almost always correct. Once the parents let go, the child could leave.

What happens there? What does the child realize? These incidents were not a matter of the parents whispering into the child's ear, "It's okay for you to go now." Besides, most of the children in question could not be said to have had any sort of consciousness left that could receive such a direct message—although that, of course, could be yet another "scientific" misreading. Nevertheless, something happened, again and again, some message was sent and received, some permission given to alter the connection. I do not say "sever" the connection, because it would seem that a link as profound as these (and all other?) parent child bonds may well not be breakable, only transmutable into a different and as yet indescribable state.

The practice of medicine, the privilege of attending the sick and the dying opens one up to a universe of reality that goes so far beyond what science can describe, even beyond what theology can grasp or articulate. There is so much more to us and our relations, to the workings of the world and the possibilities of transcendence than we can compass. The joy and, on occasion, the terror of being a doctor or a nurse lie in being exposed, time after time, to the "more" that's always there. This sense of the ineffable can bind physicians and nurses securely to the vocation of medicine, support and strengthen us in it, if we can resist the constant temptation to hide from it behind the half-truths of a superficial scientific or even religious confidence. The wonders are there to be known, but not grasped.

Chapter 11

God Will Find a Way

THIS TIME THE CALL for a bed in the P.I.C.U. came from the pediatric neurologist. There was a child in intensive care at the National Institutes of Health (N.I.H.) whose parents wanted him transferred so they could be closer to their family. The child, Jermaine Rogers, now sixteen months old, initially had been admitted to our hospital several months earlier by this neurologist because the child had been losing his developmental skills. He no longer attempted to walk and had even lost the ability to sit on his own. His age-appropriate cooing and babbling efforts at language had faded into nothing more than grunts and cries. The evaluation at that time, while it yielded no definitive diagnosis, showed with certainty that he had some sort of degenerative neurological disease that could not fail to follow the course of all similar disorders, more or less swiftly to death. Jermaine's parents, in love with this much-wanted child—their second, born twenty years after the first—could not believe this, especially in the absence of a name for the disease, something they could look up in the library to make sense of the intolerable idea that their child could not be treated and would soon die. At their request, the neurologist referred them to the N.I.H. for a second opinion, and they went gladly.

They were at the N.I.H. for months, spring to fall. There the clinicians and researchers could only confirm the original impression, although they could do so with somewhat more precision. Jermaine had an as-yet-unnamed disorder of the mitochondria, the energy system, of his nerve and muscle cells. His specific version of mitochondrial failure was thus far unique but close enough to other, also rare varieties for the prognosis to be undeniable. His nerve and muscle cells, their energy supply dwindling to zero, were dying off piecemeal, their shared functions weakened then left undone. Jermaine's muscles could no longer support him, and his nerves could not tell them to do so anyway. Even without a textbook entry for the disorder, the N.I.H. physicians had a lot to tell his parents: The inescapable consequence of this deterioration was that, sooner rather than later, Jermaine's respiratory muscles would no longer do the work of breathing for him, and, before or after that happened, his heart muscles would no longer be able to pump blood. There was nothing available, or even remotely imaginable, that medicine could offer to halt the process or to replace function, once lost. A ventilator to support his breathing, when that gave out, would only prolong the inevitable, for nothing could restore the deteriorating muscles of his heart. Even a heart transplant would not begin to solve his problems. Jermaine was going to die, probably within a few months.

However, before they said any of this to his parents, Jermaine stopped breathing, and the N.I.H. physicians, despite what they knew, intubated him and attached the tube to a ventilator to breathe for him, without having discussed the ultimate futility of that move with his parents. Now the N.I.H. staff wanted to take him off the ventilator and allow him to die. Mr. and Mrs. Rogers, although they had by now heard all that the doctors wanted them to know, refused and asked that their son be transferred back to our hospital. Thus the neurologist's request for a P.I.C.U. bed.

I groaned. To give one of the precious four P.I.C.U. beds to a child with no hope of survival (that is not what intensive care is for, I muttered into the phone) but with what promised to be an extended course of dying while his parents fought any attempts to bring the inevitable closer sounded like a nightmare. What fools had put him on the ventilator in the first place? Nothing in medical ethics requires a physician to do something futile. Cowards. Researchers without an ounce of clinical sensitivity in their brains. In my anger (but in my mind only, not aloud, fortunately), I fell back on all the usual slander of "that other hospital"— the lofty status of the N.I.H. notwithstanding—even as I knew that the same thing could well have happened, probably would have happened, at my medical center. It gave me someone to blame for what I now anticipated. But, on the other hand, there were the parents to consider: they needed not to be 500 miles away from family while this tragedy played itself out. We were their home hospital, and, like it or not, we were where they should be for this last act. "Yes, you can have the bed."

Jermaine arrived the next day, much as described. I saw him briefly as I made my rounds that afternoon and heard the nurse's report about his unresponsiveness. He needed no sedation to allow the ventilator to breathe for him; he had some reflex responses but nothing else and did not appear to be uncomfortable or in pain. His parents were described by the P.I.C.U. staff as quiet, friendly people who wanted to be with their son as much as possible, but were gracious in acceding to the requirements of the unit. The nurses' comments let me know that they saw the problem as I did and were resigned to yet another long-term, hopeless boarder, of whom there had been far too many in the P.I.C.U.

We all still carried the haunting memory of Dustin, a patient who had languished in the P.I.C.U. for more than a year because his parents' lawyers insisted there was more money to be extracted from the toy manufacturer they held responsible for his strangulation if Dustin were alive and expensive than if he were dead and no longer a financial burden. He should have been allowed to die months earlier from the pervasive hypoxic damage that had left him unaware of everything but pain, but instead he had been kept alive by all extraordinary means until he finally contracted an overwhelming sepsis that killed him quickly despite treatment. The long days of caring for him and about him had taken their toll on the staff. His parents had dealt with their grief at home; they rarely came in after the first few weeks. "Dustin" became the unit's shorthand for that which was intolerable in pediatric intensive care: intense but futile labor, intense emotional attachment that has no reasonable hope of seeing the beloved child survive, intense moral distress at the staff's helplessness in the face of powerful forces—legal, economic, egotistical, pedagogical, scientific, and so many others—that seemed to care about everything but the welfare of the child and the well-being of the workers. As the nurses told me about Jermaine, I think we all saw Dustin's ghost hovering in the background.

Two days after Jermaine was admitted, the neurologist called me. "I'd like to transfer Jermaine to your service."

Oh, great, I thought, just what I need. "Why?" I asked warily.

"I just can't work with these parents," he spat out through what sounded like clenched teeth. "They simply can't accept his diagnosis and the fact that he's going to die. They won't hear of taking him off the ventilator. They won't even let me talk about it! They're some kind of religious fanatics, you know, and they have this absurd idea that God's going to step in and heal him—and we have to keep him going until God gets around to it!"

He paused, then added with much less heat, "And . . . I think there could be some bad feeling left from when he was in here before. You know, I was the one who had to give them the diagnosis first and, well, I think they just associate me with the bad news."

I'll bet, I mused. You are not exactly famous for your charming bedside manner. Let it go and think, I chastised myself. "Yes, I'll take him. Tell the parents I'll be by later this afternoon to examine him, and then I'll come talk with them."

He signed off with a brusque "Thanks."

What have I done? I wondered. But, to tell the truth, I saw myself as being good at working with "difficult" families. I was quite sure I could convince them to let us take Jermaine off the ventilator. I even remember thinking, with a satisfied snort, "I'll have him out of there by the end of the week." How stupid. Self-righteousness is a constant temptation for those who profess medicine, for whom the pressure to be right creates too many opportunities to feign unwarranted authority or unattained skills. And it can be a most effective blinder, as I learned the hard way in this case, as in others.

I examined Jermaine thoroughly and reviewed his chart. If one could disregard the ventilator attachment and his location in an I.C.U., Jermaine looked like a peacefully sleeping, healthy, beautiful toddler, with a full head of curly dark hair, long curving eyelashes, smooth and unmarked coffee-colored skin, and an easy rise and fall of his chest with each breath. But this was a child who would neither rouse from his sleep nor shake off his posture of repose. Jermaine was not brain dead, but he was certainly absent. Although he was receiving no sedating or paralyzing medications, he responded to neither verbal nor physical stimuli, with the exception of an occasional withdrawal reflex when a finger was pinched. These reflex responses were not accompanied by grimaces or any changes in his pulse rate, so they did appear to be reflexes only and not evidence of awareness of pain. His limbs were flaccid. He had been quite stable since his return to us, requiring no changes in ventilator settings and no additional oxygen. His lungs were normal—it was his chest muscles that no longer worked. His pulse was a bit fast and his blood pressure at the lower limits of normal for his age. All was as the neurologist had described.

My conversation with Jermaine's parents was a revelation. Jermaine's parents had met in college, where they were both accounting majors. After graduation they had started a small business in a town less than thirty minutes from our hospital, where they could be close to both families. Their accounting firm had been modestly successful, such that they were able to hire a replacement for Mrs. Rogers while she was with Jermaine at the N.I.H.; Mr. Rogers had stayed behind to continue running the business. Their enforced separation seemed to have been one of the major reasons for their requesting Jermaine's transfer back to us—that and the presence of their large extended family back home, plus a church community in which they were deeply involved. They had found it impossible to live through such a crisis so far from all that held them together as a family and as individuals.

They treasured their older child, now in her last year of college, but had always wanted more children. It had not seemed to be in the cards until the "miraculous" pregnancy with Jermaine happened, long after they had stopped hoping for another child. He was a beautiful, healthy baby who was precocious in his development, ready to walk at nine months, and generous in his affections. Then came the incomprehensible changes: his attention turned inward, his smiles fewer, and he showed no interest in standing up—followed by the day when he could no longer sit without support. That was the signal to them that he was not just taking a breather from his accelerated developmental course. He was moving backward, losing the skills he had already mastered so easily.

We discussed the process of diagnosis and what it had been like for them to hear the verdict. They briefly mentioned that the neurologist's abruptness had exacerbated the pain of his message, but were at pains to assure me that they had never doubted his explanations and prognosis. Their insistence on a second opinion had to do with their perception of their obligations to Jermaine, and to God, rather than with any lack of trust in the neurologist's competence or truthfulness. They understood and accepted the information he had given them, as they did the more detailed confirmation from the N.I.H. doctors—they could, in fact, tell me more about it than I had already gleaned. However, they did not believe that the medical pronouncements were the last word on Jermaine. Their faith, the central motif of their lives, assured them that God was in charge of prognoses and could effect a cure, or some other form of recovery, despite the hopeless picture presented by the medical experts.[1] They did not know whether God *would* do so in this case—they were far from blindly optimistic—but they were quite sure the decision was God's to make and not theirs or ours.

After that first discussion, we parted amicably. I had a lot to think about. I felt great respect and admiration for their strength, their understanding, and, yes, the solidity of their belief. They were not the "fanatics" the neurologist had declared them to be, not by my understanding of the word. They were intelligent, reasonable people, facing an unfathomable grief with courage and steadfastness, while remaining faithful to the truth of their lives. I began to reconstrue my obligations as not only to care for Jermaine but also to honor his parents as they found their own way through this dreadful upheaval.

Little changed over the next few weeks, with the exception of the growing restlessness of some of my colleagues. The head of the adult medical I.C.U., the unit that got the P.I.C.U.'s "overflow" when its four beds were full, as was usually the case, called me daily to quiz me about my apparent commitment to providing futile care in the P.I.C.U. As he intoned, more than once, we are under no moral or legal obligation to provide futile care (conveniently begging the basic question of how to define *futile*). He urged me to take Jermaine off the ventilator, to let him die and free up the P.I.C.U.'s allotment of scarce resources. I understood his point all too well; I had often been the one making the same argument to other physicians with patients in the P.I.C.U. who, in my view, should not be there. Dustin's case had been a paradigm of futility and frustration. But at the same time, I continued to talk with Jermaine's parents, and I knew I could not make a unilateral decision to stop life support. There was work going on here that was not futile.

In one of my many conversations with Jermaine's parents, after we had come to know each other better, I heard more of their beliefs about God's willingness to intervene directly in people's lives, to heal just at the time when there seems no hope of healing. Because they had been so honest with me about their faith, I thought I could say something of what I believed. This was by no means a usual practice for me, but in this situation I felt sharply the mismatch between their giving and my receiving. They had been open with me, trusting that I would respect what they said and neither turn away nor try to overcome their theology with my science. I could no longer be only a blank sounding board. Tentatively, I ventured out.

"I also believe that God is involved somehow, even intensely involved, in our illnesses and our healings," I said. "But I just can't believe God plays games with us, especially about something as painful as this. I mean, if God were going to cure Jermaine, I think it would have happened long before now. I don't think God would wait until Jermaine's brain and body are so terribly damaged and you have gone through these months of agony, just to pull it out at the end so it looks like an even bigger miracle. It would have been a miracle seven months ago. Why wait?"

They nodded their understanding of my position; I suspect they had been there several times over. Mr. Rogers responded: "That may be true. You may be right. But we just don't know, do we? We don't know what God may be going to do. And our job, while we're waiting to see what he'll do, is to make sure we don't place any obstacles in his way. If we take Jermaine off that ventilator, we take away from God any chance of his acting. We can't do that."

I began to see more clearly then an idea that had been taking shape in my mind over the years I had been caring for critically ill children. There was a definite limit—its location not always distinct, but the fact of the boundary certain nonetheless—to what I could do for patients in my care. My knowledge and skill were of primary importance and had to be used well on their behalf, but, once all that could and should be done was done, the children would survive or they would not. The families, however, especially the parents, would without question outlive their child's illness. The quality of *their* survival—what the rest of their lives would be like after the critical event, with or without a surviving child—had something to do with how I worked with them during the crisis. In the case of Jermaine's parents, in particular, I realized that, although Jermaine would surely die (I still did not believe God would stage a last-minute restoration), it was of central importance to his parents' future that they be able to remember that in the midst of the struggle they had remained faithful to Jermaine and to God, according to their understanding of what such fidelity required.

During that conversation, or perhaps another, I found that they were familiar with the concept of brain death. Further, were Jermaine brain dead, they would interpret that to be sufficient evidence that God did not intend to heal him, and they then would not oppose taking him off life support. That interchange led me to ask them whether there were situations other than brain death that might also count as reliable signs that Jermaine's death was within God's will. Puzzled, they asked for examples. Well, I posited, he could develop an overwhelming infection, as happens to children on ventilators and intravenous feedings, that might outstrip the power of any antibiotic we have available. Yes, they thought, that would be convincing. If the antibiotics could not stop the infection, there would be no point in doing anything more, no point in trying to resuscitate him if his heart stopped because of the sepsis.

And then, I said, there is his heart. We had talked before about the evidence we already had that Jermaine's disease was sapping the strength of his heart muscle. His rapid pulse and low-normal blood pressure had been the first indications of a heart trying harder but accomplishing less. Subsequent studies had confirmed that his heart was becoming as flabby and unresponsive to nerve impulses as had the rest of his musculature. We had put him on a medication to support his blood pressure, but it provided only slight improvement. I had not expected, nor led his parents to expect, that it would make much difference—thus, I could justify its use to myself, believing that it could not significantly prolong the inevitable but would honor his parents' desires for treatment. We had discussed the likelihood that Jermaine's death would come that way, as heart failure that we could not overcome. Now I asked if that too would count as evidence that God was not going to work a miracle for Jermaine. Yes, they nodded, certainly. They agreed that resuscitative efforts were not to be used if Jermaine's heart failed. No "code," no chest compressions, no frantic attempts to infuse energy into a heart that could no longer use it.

It was only a few days after we had that conversation that Jermaine's heart gave up the struggle. That morning his blood pressure began dropping steadily, despite the medication still flowing into his veins. His parents had not yet come in to visit. I called them at home to describe what was happening. They knew what it meant and decided to stay home and gather their family and friends around them while I kept them informed by phone. Within the hour, Jermaine's heart went into "electromechanical dissociation," a condition in which the nerves stimulate the heart appropriately, as indicated by the electrocardiogram (E.K.G.), but the heart muscle fails to respond by contracting. Despite electrical activity mimicking a normal E.K.G., there is no pulse, no pumping action by the heart, no flow of blood through the body. In Jermaine's case, this was the final degeneration. He died quietly, almost ten weeks after his return from the N.I.H.

I called his parents to tell them that Jermaine was dead. They thanked me briefly and hung up. They called back later to give information about the funeral home they had chosen. I never heard from them again, but I have never forgotten what they taught me. Nor have I ever doubted that keeping Jermaine on the ventilator was the right thing to do. Had there been any evidence that he was suffering, it would have been a different matter. I cannot be certain how things would have turned out in that event, although I imagine I would have been called on, by his parents and by my own sense of obligation, to do all possible to relieve that suffering before using it as a trumping argument for stopping his life support. Were his suffering ultimately unrelievable, I like to think they would have agreed not to force Jermaine to stay in his tortured body. They, I suspect, know the scriptures better than I: God does not test us beyond our power to endure, but always provides a way out.

I have said that I realized, in working with Jermaine's parents, that the nature of my encounters with them could have some effect on the quality of their survival of such a terrible loss. I still believe this to be true, although, as is the case with most of the families I have known, I do not know how their lives after Jermaine's death played out. I hope they have continued to find the strength and consolation, in each other and in their beliefs, that carried them through his protracted dying. Their faithfulness—to Jermaine, to God, to themselves, and to their extended families—stands as a lasting reminder to me of the complexity of what we do and whom we touch in medicine and of the truth that, in virtually every serious medical intervention, there is more than one "patient" whose life is at stake.

PART III

Waiting

Attend: III. To wait for, await, expect

How could you permit yourself to breathe, let alone laugh or sleep or eat well, if you were unable to imagine how hard another person's life was?

—Jonathan Franzen, *The Corrections*

In part III, the combination of my continued growth in the role of doctor and the nature of primary care encounters makes for longer, more pensive, quieter accounts, in which reflection becomes a more integral part of each story. The level of detail has increased not only because the relationships last longer and the events are closer in time to my recording of them but also because I had become better at paying attention, at noticing and incorporating what I saw and heard into my understandings of my patients' lives.

These stories are full of my waiting—for the next visit, the next phone call, the next need to be voiced. Waiting, of course, implies long stretches of time when nothing happens or, rather, when what is happening is occurring somewhere else. If, after the concentrated action in most of the previous stories, these narratives sound fragmented, episodic, patchy—flashes of lives that, for the most part, are lived offstage and unknown to me between these recorded encounters—that's the way it was. In primary care, the claim that medical encounters represent intersections of the doctor's life with the lives of patients and families requires no argument. We do not travel the same road for even an hour, and the times when our paths cross may be weeks, months, or years apart. I can say more about Janet (chapter 14) from age nine to seventeen than I ever could about Mickey, whom I knew intensely for only six months of her thirteenth year. However, my apparently copious knowledge of Janet, like the details I can offer about the other primary care patients I describe here, came in fits and starts in the widely spaced glimpses of events and personality that sporadic visits to clinic afforded.

It is an enormous privilege to have known patients and their families as well as I have. I have known them in their pain and distress, their joys and successes, their denials and confusions, their strong days and their weak days. With time and attention, I could learn to tell one kind of day from the other and even to know something about why they were that way and what might be done to help. But no doctor is, can be, or should be even close to omniscient about a patient's life. We speak much of confidentiality in medicine—far less of privacy—but privacy is an important moral category to remember in dealing with the manifest incompleteness of these stories. For example, Janet's life is her own, and she, like my other patients, more or less willingly allowed me to see parts of it, even to participate in writing occasional paragraphs on widely separated pages in the encyclopedic tome of her existence, but we shall not be reading the whole work.

It can be fairly argued, on the evidence of the stories in part III, that the outcome of my search for balance settled on the side of "overinvolvement" or, at least, what many in the medical profession would label as such. I frankly confess not only to regularly being deeply involved with patients and their families but also to believing that there is much to be said for it, for being fully aware of and responsive to what is happening at the intersection of my patient's life and my life.

I believe that medical professionals, in general, are prone to overdiagnosing overinvolvement. A colleague of mine often reminds me that we do a fairly good job in medical education of teaching students, mostly by example, how to maintain professional distance; we are much less accomplished in teaching them how to negotiate the levels of intimacy that so often arise within patient–physician encounters and that can be so important for the well-being of both parties. This skewed pedagogical emphasis renders us inordinately wary of emotional engagement with patients, perceiving it as an unmapped swamp of leechlike need and distorted vision. We are therefore quick to label almost any level of meaningful absorption in the interlocking patient-physician narrative as excessive, as *over*involvement (and, ipso facto, unprofessional), while being significantly less concerned about the reverse problem of *under*involvement. With due respect to the importance of retaining the ability to make necessary professional judgments by avoiding the paralysis that deep emotional entanglement may cause, I believe that underinvolvement is much more likely to result in mistaken decisions, misunderstandings, and miscommunications. A determined resistance to being truly engaged with—and raptly attentive to—patients and families creates a more effective paralysis of judgment than does virtually any degree of willingness to be moved by their predicaments.

It is possible, certainly, to be too involved, to cross over an invisible, shifting boundary into a place where the tasks of doctoring become difficult or impossible to perform appropriately. The difficulty is in knowing where, in any given situation, that boundary lies. Discerning the limits is a matter of attention and experience, the latter far more effectively gained by straying close to the edge rather than by keeping a "safe" distance. My encounters with Mickey and her family (chapter 4), for example, helped me discern my place with Jennie and her family (chapter 7), ten years later. These cumulative experiences helped shape my engagement with the Morris family (chapter 13), another fifteen years into my career. To tell the truth, even if it were possible, I would not go back and decrease my level of involvement with any of the patients and families I have known, but there are many with whom I wish I had been more closely engaged, to whom I wish I had paid more attention, for their sakes and for mine.

Chapter 12

Presumptuous Empathy

ON MY WAY DOWN the hall to the "residents' room" where we did all our paperwork, I was stopped by Lynn Foster, whose children were patients in our clinic practice.

"Dr. Mohrmann, could I talk with you before you go in to see Carla?"

"Oh, Carla's here today?" Carla was one of her daughters.

"Yeah. I want you to talk with her too, but I need some time with you first."

"Sure. Is it okay if a resident goes in to see her while we talk?"

"Oh, that's fine, but . . . well, I need to talk with you, you know, privately."

I knew Lynn fairly well, having seen her and her children several times for a variety of reasons, none out of the ordinary. She was a white woman in her mid- to late thirties, always stylishly coifed and dressed, her fingernails carefully painted in colors to match her outfits. Lynn had three children. Michelle, now twenty years old, had a child of her own, one-year-old Tommy, whom she brought to us for his well-child care. The other two children were Brian, a fifteen-year-old boy seen mostly in a specialty clinic for management of his allergies, and Carla, now thirteen. Later I learned that Lynn had another child, her oldest, a man in his early twenties, who was by this time married and living about an hour away with his wife and baby daughter.

I gave Carla's chart to one of the residents and explained to him that I would be talking with Ms. Foster while he got Carla's history. I cannot now recall the reason for Carla's visit; it may well have been some minor symptom used by her mother as a ticket to get her in for a talking-to. Lynn and I went into an empty examination room, and I closed the door.

"So, how can I help you?" I began.

She immediately spilled out her concerns about Carla. Recently a young man had moved in next door; Carla was becoming very interested in him and, apparently, he in her. They were spending a lot of time in their adjoining backyards talking over the fence, and Lynn was pretty sure they had been seeing each other elsewhere too, although Carla would not admit to it or, more precisely, would refuse to respond to questions on that topic. The young man was twenty-two years old. Lynn's attempts to discuss the situation with Carla, which usually included telling her point-blank that this man was too old for her and that she could not date him, quickly terminated in screams, tears, and slammed doors. She did not know how to reach Carla about her concerns and wanted me to talk with her.

"You know how it is with girls and their mothers. She just won't listen to me, but she'll listen to you, I'm sure."

I was not so certain.

I asked Lynn if she had talked with the young man and made sure he knew that Carla was only thirteen, even, if necessary, reminding him that sexual relations with Carla—which was clearly what Lynn was concerned about—would be a crime, putting him on notice that she was watching and would not hesitate to call the police. She had indeed let him know that Carla was much too young for him, but, as Lynn told it, he had blown her off, saying it was up to Carla to choose whom she spent time with. His willful irresponsibility heightened Lynn's sense of urgency and prompted her to seek help at the clinic. She had made the appointment with me because, she said, Carla really respected me and would listen to what I told her. Oh, good. What now? Anything I said to Carla may or may not have the desired effect, but of more concern to me at the moment was helping Lynn find ways to reopen communication with her daughter. They had always been close, and Carla had seemed to trust her mother. Was this just a dramatic beginning to her teenage years and the inevitable changes in their relationship? Lynn used to be so confident in her handling of the children; she had had plenty of experience dealing with the storms of adolescence. Why was this one such a stopper for her?

I was at a loss to know where to go with this and also puzzled by the forceful passion of Lynn's reaction to what was going on. To buy time, and with the half-formed idea that it might help Lynn to remember what she knew about the angst and emotional lability of this age group, I asked her, "What was it like for you at thirteen?"

She was quiet for a long moment, looking down at her hands. When she looked up at me to answer my question, tears were rolling down her cheeks. Things had been rough for her at thirteen. She described to me what her childhood had been like in her chaotic, difficult family. The details were, and are, painful and intensely private; she had not discussed them with anyone before. At the age of thirteen, Lynn had run off with a twenty-one-year-old man—"The first one who came along," she said with a grim half-smile—in order to get away from home. She had her first child when she was fourteen.

I put my hand on her arm and sat quietly with her, absorbing the pain and grief of her story. "I'm sorry, Lynn. I'm so sorry. How awful for you." Or some such inarticulate words that one offers when there is nothing adequate to be said, something just to acknowledge reception of the enormity of it and to clarify the silence as one not of disapproval and revulsion but of sorrow and respect.

"And to have held it all inside all these years. Have you never talked with anyone about all this? Maybe your sister? After all, she was living there too."

"I just couldn't. Besides, what good would it do now? And my sister"—here she snorted in disgust—"I tried to talk with her once, and she denied everything. She said I was lying and just trying to make excuses for getting pregnant so young. We don't get along so well anyway. Never have."

As we sat there, moving between meditative silence and spontaneous brief dialogues, her thoughts seemed to shift back toward Carla. After a while, Lynn said, "I see. That's why this is so hard."

Together we acknowledged the potent fear and passionate refusal that accompanied her perception that parts of her past were threatening to be replayed in her daughter's life, the child she would protect from everything. Lynn revealed a little about what it had been like to have a child at fourteen, another at sixteen, and then to have been abandoned by their father. There was another man after that, the father of Brian and Carla, but he had left too, at which point she had "sworn off men," in her words. For most of her twenty-plus years of child rearing, she had been a single mother, without a high school diploma, enough money to go around, or a family she could turn to for support. It terrified her to think of Carla putting herself in a similarly precarious position. So, she realized, her terror had rendered her incapable of coping well with the threat that the young man next door represented. Thus she reacted in furious alarm, understandably translated by Carla as an unreasonable attempt at control.

"Can you talk to Carla about why this is so hard?"

"Oh, I don't think so. Maybe later, not now."

We considered ways of reaching Carla with Lynn's well-founded concerns, ways of handling the situation, legally if it came to that, as well as emotionally. Plus, Lynn's long-festering wounds needed attention, especially now that she had stripped the old bandages off. I strongly encouraged her to seek counseling and gave her the names of some therapists. I told her I would talk with Carla, and I suggested another visit the following week to continue the conversation with each of them. She readily agreed.

I saw Carla alone after that, the resident having dealt with her medical complaint appropriately, and tried to present her mother's trepidation in a way she might be able to hear and appreciate, but without divulging what I now knew about Lynn's past. I spoke in general terms of a mother's wish that her children not suffer the privations their parents had known, if possible, and more specifically about how difficult it had been for her mother to rear her children as a solitary teen mother and how that might fuel her fears for Carla. Carla's response, of course, was that she had no intention of becoming a mother nor, for that matter, of having sex with this man; he was just a friend. So I talked about what twenty-two-year-old male friends can ask, or demand, of thirteen-year-old girls and about the importance of protecting herself—and I told her about the law and her mother's willingness to use it. She was stunned to learn that her new friend would soon be in jail if they had sexual relations, that the law did not consider her old enough to consent, no matter how mature she felt herself to be.

"Not fair," the universal cry of outraged children, erupted from her.

"Fair or not, that's the way it is. Be careful with this, Carla. Don't get in over your head."

She pouted and nodded, eager to be gone.

This encounter had happened on a Tuesday afternoon. The following Friday morning, I opened the newspaper at breakfast. There on the front page was a picture of a demolished car and an article about a terrible wreck on a rainy county road Thursday afternoon that had killed three young people and left one infant badly injured. I read through the article, mildly interested in such a dreadful but distant event, until I hit the paragraph that identified the victims. Michelle, Brian, and Carla Foster, all dead—and Tommy in intensive care. My dear God. I reread it to see if I could be mistaken. I was not. As soon as I got to the clinic that morning, I found the nurses. Yes, they had seen the article. Yes, they were our patients. Yes. All three.

Frances, the exceptional master of records in our clinic, who had worked there for years and knew everyone by sight and by medical record number, saw Lynn in the hospital cafeteria a few days later. After a long hug, Lynn explained that she was at the hospital day and night with Tommy in the P.I.C.U. By the time Frances saw Lynn, Tommy was out of danger, and his mother, aunt, and uncle had been buried side by side near the farm where Lynn had spent her childhood.

Tommy improved rapidly and was transferred within a week to the children's rehabilitation unit, where he stayed for a month or so. I received reports of his progress—Lynn had taken immediate custody of Tommy and designated me as his primary care doctor—informing me that therapists were working on strengthening his right arm and leg, weakened by the blow to the left side of his brain, and that he was getting steadily stronger.

After Tommy left the hospital, I saw him in the clinic with some frequency, both to assess his progress (which was consistently good; within a year of his time in the P.I.C.U., he had no apparent motor impairment or other overt evidence of residual brain damage) and to give Lynn the opportunity to talk. It had become clear on our first few visits after the catastrophe that she had few people she could talk with about what had happened and how she was dealing with it, while taking on the care of an active toddler at the same time. Her mother seemed too wrapped up in the loss of her grandchildren to tend to Lynn's need for comfort, and Lynn was not willing to add her own infinite grief to her mother's burden—plus, she was never completely at ease with her family or in her childhood home.

I had hoped the gravity of the situation would help reconcile Lynn with her sister, but, in fact, things were worse than ever between them. In a particularly grim trick of fate, Lynn's sister and her husband, on their way to the same event the children were headed toward, had been one of the first cars to happen upon the accident. At first, Lynn told me only about the pain of her sister's using this experience to insist that her own suffering, as an eyewitness, took precedence over Lynn's, creating a bizarre and ghoulish competition for the sympathy of friends and family members. This was a contest in which Lynn was neither able nor willing to participate, and she was angered both by her sister's commandeering the tragedy for her own uses and by her extended family's failure to see through the ploy and keep their focus on Lynn, the one who had sustained the primary loss.

It took a bit longer for Lynn to tell me the other reason her sister's presence at the scene of the wreck was such a barrier between them. Her sister had been determined to tell Lynn—repeatedly and despite Lynn's pleas that she not—every detail of what she had witnessed. Now Lynn was torn between the stories and images that intensified her suffering and the testimonies that helped ease it. She was particularly haunted by the narrative picture she had been given of Michelle's final moments. According to Lynn's sister, when they arrived at the scene, they found Michelle impaled on the steering column but still alive, semiconscious and moaning Tommy's name. Lynn's brother-in-law, holding the injured but obviously alive Tommy in his arms, brought him over to Michelle's side to assure her that he was all right. Michelle looked up and saw her living son, smiled, and died. Lynn was wracked by the unwanted, but now indelible, mental picture of her daughter pierced and dying, and at the same time soothed by the thought that Michelle's dying thoughts had been of Tommy. The image had given her nightmares, but it also provided the basis for a story she would tell Tommy again and again about how much his mother had loved him. Lynn's ambivalence about her sister's presence at the children's deaths was heightened by the other tale she had brought to her: Carla, seated in the backseat of the car beside Tommy's car seat, appeared to have thrown herself across Tommy in a spontaneous and desperate attempt to protect him. One of the police officers at the scene said that she had saved Tommy's life by doing that. Lynn clung to this interpretation of the position in which Carla's body had been found as evidence of her daughter's innate goodness and as a sign that Tommy was fated to survive.

During that first year after the accident, Lynn told me about what she was doing to make sure Tommy did not forget Michelle, his "real" mother. She had set up a shrine of sorts for the three children—a table with their photographs, some items of meaning to them and to her, and candles. This she did for herself, to create a place of intense remembrance where she could concentrate and briefly lay down her unrelenting pain. In addition to creating the shrine, she had placed pictures of Michelle around the house, especially in Tommy's room. Lynn told me she often used those pictures almost as storybooks, holding Tommy in her lap as she showed him photographs of Michelle and told him stories about how much Michelle had loved him. She taught him to point to the pictures and say "Mommy," because Tommy, being a very young child, had started calling Lynn "Mama" soon after his return from the hospital. He had been too young before Michelle's death to have settled on a grandmotherly name for Lynn, so the universal baby "mmm" sound that comes to attach itself to mother became spontaneously, understandably reassigned to Lynn. She accepted the honorific gladly, while still insisting that this toddler recognize the photographs of Michelle as his "real" mother. Lynn became Tommy's legal mother by adopting him outright. His father, a young Mexican immigrant who had been only minimally involved in Tommy's life in his first year, readily signed over his parental rights to allow the adoption to take place.

Lynn had her problems with Tommy. By several months after the accident, he seemed to have fully recovered neurologically, looking and acting much like any two-year-old boy. But he began having occasional episodes—"little fits" she called them—sometimes during play, sometimes awakening him from sleep, that sounded like a cross between night terrors and seizures, in which he would stare, scream or cry, and be unreachable for a few minutes. I could not say whether he had recurring memories of the accident, as Lynn feared, that could terrorize his dreams and startle him in the midst of his daily activities. He had been given anticonvulsant medication during his hospital stay, because of the risk of seizures with a head injury as severe as his, but it had been stopped before his discharge. Did he need it now? After some testing and consultation with neurologists, we decided to restart the anticonvulsant, not least because Lynn found the "fits" so unnerving. He stayed on it for about a year, during which the episodes gradually decreased in frequency, from several a week to one every few weeks, then disappeared altogether by the time he outgrew his medication dosage. We stopped the drug, and the episodes did not return. We were never sure what they portended, if anything.

Probably more disheartening for both Lynn and me were her difficulties with disciplining Tommy. This was a major topic of discussion at his clinic visits. During each visit a pediatric resident would go in first to take the history and do a physical examination. Lynn did not offer her full story to the residents who examined Tommy, nor did they think to ask for such a tale. Who would? So they would return and describe her to me as they saw her: an older mother, abnormally attached to her only child and hopelessly incapable of disciplining him. I would then tell them what had happened to her children, and they could then perhaps begin to understand what Lynn readily acknowledged to me: that she could not consistently correct Tommy's behavior—could not feed him anything but the bacon and french fries that were all he would accept for months, could not train him to use the toilet or drink from a cup against his will—because he was all she had, and she could not risk another loss.

I would gently remind Lynn of the skills she had acquired while rearing her children, the hard-won realization that disciplining a child would not cause her to lose him, but that, on the contrary, her reluctance to help him become "civilized" put both of them at risk for later losses. She never argued these points with me, just listened silently, nodding at me and smiling at her son/grandson, busy with his exploration of the examining room. But when the actual tests of her resolve arose, as they did daily, she still found herself unable to abide his infant anger or counter his stubborn demands.

At most of Tommy's clinic visits, I spent time encouraging Lynn to get counseling of some sort, both for her own grief and anger and for her problems with enforcing discipline. I offered a variety of possibilities for individual therapy, or counseling for her and Tommy together, or participation in groups of bereaved parents. She always listened politely, agreed with me wholeheartedly, and did nothing. I believed I understood her reluctance to seek psychological support of any sort. What had happened in her life was so overwhelming, she would naturally be less than eager to confront it again in therapy. Plus—this was my basic reasoning about it—she had never dealt with her own disastrous childhood. The one time she had talked about it had been followed within days by the deaths of her children. How could she bring herself to expose that subject again, much less explore it? I was content with what I thought was my sensitive grasp of the situation and unaware of the extent to which my "empathic" understanding, my construal of what must be the case for Lynn, was determined by my own perspectives and experiences. So I just kept gently prodding her from time to time to take care of herself too.

The time came when the problems with Tommy's behavior became intolerable for her. She, along with the physical therapists and speech therapists who continued to work with him after his brain injury, wanted him to be in preschool for the developmental stimulation it offered and the opportunity to play with other children his age. Not only did she fear that he would not tolerate the separation from her, but she also knew that preschool required that he be out of diapers, off the bottle, and used to trying foods that were not on his list of particular preferences. All the battles she had been avoiding were looming, and she did not know how to face them. I knew I could help her to some degree with techniques I had learned over the years for getting around recalcitrant toddlers, but the scope of the issue went way beyond behavior modification tricks. I pushed counseling once more, this time suggesting that the two of them go together and focus solely on the parenting issues, if the rest were still too painful for her to deal with. But she resisted again, and this time I had the sense to ask her why. What was keeping her from seeing a counselor?

Lynn readily explained it to me, so readily that I later wondered if she had just been waiting for me to ask. She was quite sure that in counseling of any sort she would lose her always-tenuous control on her grief and break down in front of the therapist. She believed that the therapist would see her as emotionally unstable and therefore unfit to be a mother for Tommy, who would then be taken away from her. I was astonished. It had never entered my mind that her resistance to therapy had to do with fears of losing Tommy (in retrospect, I am mostly astonished at my blindness), not with fears of confronting her own past. I immediately assured her that no therapist I knew would see her grief as emotional instability or see her as an unfit parent because of it. Furthermore, she had legally adopted Tommy, and he could not be snatched away from her on such flimsy grounds.

"Oh," she said, "I didn't know that. Sure, I'll make the appointment."

She did, and the counseling made a significant difference in her ability to care for Tommy, who entered preschool just a few months later, without diaper or bottle. If I had looked beyond my "highly empathic" assumptions earlier and found out from her, rather than from my own suppositions, how she comprehended the situation, perhaps she would have gotten that help much sooner.

Empathy, a characteristic sought for and praised when found in health care workers, is a complex concept with significant potential for misuse. The urge to enter into—by listening, paying attention, being present—a patient's experience of suffering, so that one may not only offer appropriate aid but also, in some sense, share the burden of the pain, is certainly a good impulse, to be encouraged in and modeled for doctors and nurses in training. The risk of misuse comes with the medical professional's assessment that, once having grasped something of the patient's truth, there is no more to know and thus steps can be taken based on one's (necessarily partial) understanding rather than on the explicit directions of the patient.

The truth is that, no matter how intimate the bond I have with a patient, no matter how skilled I may become at seeing through my patient's eyes and entering into his or her experience of suffering, I am still a separate person. It is still Dr. Mohrmann, with all my own life experiences, education, understandings of the world—construals of health and the body and what is and is not important in life—trying to look through the patient's eyes. It is my interpretive mechanisms that are processing what I see when I try to look at events from the patient's point of view.

That is, it is one thing to be able, after careful listening and observation, to say, "I understand what you've let me know about how you feel," and to let that understanding deepen and guide one's relationship with the patient from then on. My rapport with Lynn Foster was significantly shaped by what she had allowed me to know about her life and its exigencies. There were times when she had only to raise her eyebrows and flash me a penetrating glance when, say, speaking of a visit to her mother or an encounter with her sister to tap into the reservoir of comprehension we shared. However, it is quite another thing, a dangerous and fundamentally immoral move, to proceed from such an understanding, important as it is, to the claim "I know how you feel"—surely the one statement that should be forbidden to all medical professionals. From that false claim it is but an easy slide to an even more perilous assertion: "Therefore, I know what you want (or need)." This is empathy's imperialistic proclivity, and those who wish to be truly understanding, empathic physicians, nurses, or therapists of any sort must be constantly on guard against its perversion of the good impulse to provide attentive care. I learned this, cumulatively and over many years, from my patients and their families who, like Lynn Foster, quietly revealed to me my presumptuousness and its consequences.

There was still so much I did not know about Lynn and her life. I had learned, after her children's deaths, that she had one surviving child, her oldest. By the way she spoke of him, I gathered they were estranged. He had come to the funeral for his siblings but, she told me, had spent more time with the other relatives than with her. In fact, she said, "He pretty much ignored me." He visited Lynn's mother and sister frequently, but rarely came to see Lynn. What was that about? He was the child she had borne at fourteen. What kind of mother had she been able to be for him? Did he even live with her during his childhood, or perhaps with her mother instead? There were corners of Lynn's life I was not invited to see, facets of her experience to which I had no clue. I did learn that, with time and perhaps as a side effect of great tragedy, her relationship with her surviving son softened, and I began hearing of more contact with them, especially with her granddaughter. Lynn called me a few times with medical questions about her and, on one occasion, brought her daughter-in-law and granddaughter to have me check the child for some problem. Lynn's relationship with her firstborn was, for the most part, a hidden story. I can add these few details to this story, but I do not know whether or how they fit within the narrative as whole.

Lynn's chronic fears of losing Tommy were intensified, when he was four and five years old, by threats from his father, Juan. Lynn, although not required to by law, had allowed Juan liberal visiting privileges over the years. She told me that she wanted Tommy to know his father, so he would not have to suffer the loss of both his parents. She had tried to help Juan in his own unstable life, including supporting his developing relationship with another woman, even to the point of holding their wedding in her own home with Tommy in attendance. But soon after Juan's marriage things began to change.

Juan and his wife had asked to have Tommy with them most weekends, to which Lynn agreed because Tommy seemed to enjoy being with them. However, Juan also began badgering her for permission to take his son to see his relatives in Mexico. Lynn consistently refused, fearing that, once in Mexico, Tommy might not be allowed to return, and she would be powerless to retrieve him. While this wrangle with Juan was going on, Tommy made some ambiguous but disturbing remarks that suggested he was being mistreated in some way during his weekend time with Juan and his wife, and he began to resist going to their house. Tommy's physical examination was normal and his stories jumbled, but the concerns were real enough—as was Tommy's now-adamant refusal to go to Juan's house—for Lynn to stop the weekend visits. Juan could see Tommy, but only with Lynn present.

Juan hired a lawyer to help him overturn his previous abdication of parental rights, based on claims that he had been too young to know what he was doing and that all the proceedings had been in English, which he did not understand. Lynn's lawyer, who had also handled the previous legal work of adoption, was able to demonstrate effectively, from the records and from witnesses' testimony, that Juan was over the age of legal majority at the time, had had things fully explained to him—in Spanish as well as in English—and thus had no factual basis for claiming he had been snookered out of his parental rights. The court agreed and specifically included in its decision concurrence with Lynn's fear that Juan's desire to take Tommy to Mexico was a ploy to get the child out of United States jurisdiction, as well as with her decision not to allow Juan and his wife unaccompanied visits with Tommy. After the court decision, Juan seemed to lose all interest in Tommy—Lynn was convinced it was because his wife had become pregnant—and may have moved back to Mexico. In any case, he disappeared from their lives. Tommy, fortunately, seemed more relieved than disturbed by this change as, of course, was Lynn, who was happy to see an end to a long year's worth of anxiety.

During the time that the duel with Juan was at its height, Lynn's boyfriend had moved in with her and Tommy. She had been dating Chuck for several months and seemed happier than I had seen her in a very long time. He was an auto mechanic, a little older than Lynn, and seemed to adore not only her but Tommy, an impression I formed for myself when he accompanied them for a routine clinic visit. Chuck and Tommy got on beautifully together, with Chuck taking to his paternal role eagerly and competently. Chuck could discipline Tommy in ways Lynn still could not, apparently without being unduly harsh or using physical force, something Lynn would never have allowed. Soon the answering machine at the house heralded the formation of their family: "You've reached the home of Lynn, Chuck, and Tommy." Tommy was now in kindergarten, having successfully worked his way through preschool, enjoying his peers and his new skills—and still, sometimes, looking at Michelle's picture and remembering to call her "Mommy."

Chapter 13

Bridging the Distance

IN RETROSPECT, my first exchange with the Morris family—much like that first afternoon's conference with Lynn Foster—although memorable in its own right, gave no hint of what lay in store in the years to come. A medical student had been in to see a four-year-old boy for some common complaint and presented the patient to me. The student had had some problems understanding the history of the illness as reported by the boy's father (or, he mused, might this man be his grandfather?), but thought the child was fine and in no need of medication or intervention. I went back to the examining room with him to see them—and can still vividly recall my first sight of Mr. Morris and Kevin. Mr. Morris, who was sitting in the chair closest to the door, cocked his head, squinted up at me as though the sun were in his eyes, and offered a wide, crooked grin as I entered the room. He had on a knit watch cap in bright orange—"blaze" orange, required wear for hunters—pulled low on his forehead; stiff strands of gray and brown hair protruded like a thorny halo from the cap's edge. His face was gaunt, deeply lined, ruddy, and whiskery, his thin body clothed in a plaid flannel shirt and jeans, both appearing remarkably dirty. His hands rested atop a cane that was planted on the floor between his feet, which were shod in work boots caked with dried red mud. He looked like a stereotype of backwoods Appalachia.

Mr. Morris's four-year-old son, Kevin, squirmed in the chair to his father's right. (I soon confirmed that Mr. Morris was indeed his father; although he looked at least sixty years old, I believe he was in his early forties at our first meeting.) Kevin cocked his head and squinted up at me in a precise caricature of his father's pose, but for the fact that he scowled fiercely. There were smudges of dirt on his face, and his jeans and torn T-shirt matched his father's for grime. The room was redolent of body odor, wood smoke, and a sort of earthiness.

I introduced myself in my usual generically friendly manner and shook Mr. Morris's hand. I said something welcoming to Kevin who, once my attention was directed at him, glowered more seriously, held his balled-up fists in front of his face, gave a deep growl, and then belligerently and forcefully made several jabs with his right index finger toward the door of the room, each thrust of his finger accompanied by another grunt. Message received: Get out. His father chuckled and beamed down on the little boy with proud affection. Hmm.

I sat down beside Kevin, facing the two of them, and asked Mr. Morris a few questions to corroborate and expand the student's history. I soon found myself agreeing with the student: this was rough going. Mr. Morris's answers often seemed to bear little relation to the question. My attempts to encourage him to relate the story in his own fashion evoked a single sentence, which could be loosely translated as "He's sick, needs medicine." Throughout our "conversation," Kevin watched me intensely from under lowered brows, kept his fists at the ready, and emitted an intermittent low warning rumble, disconcertingly like a dog held back by his master from attacking an enemy. An interesting encounter, this.

Not surprisingly, Kevin refused to get up on the exam table when I asked him to do so. That is, he treated that request the way he had responded to my every overture: the rumble deepened and spread to a snarl, teeth (not very healthy teeth, I could see) bared, fists coming up again. Some preschoolers enjoy playing guard dog and can be engaged in talking about the role, even giggling about it. Not so with Kevin. He was too deep in the part to respond to my recognition of his role play in any way other than as a dog. I glanced at his father, my brows raised in a silent query. Mr. Morris smiled ingratiatingly at me, with that boys-will-be-boys look of fond parental helplessness that pediatricians dread, and wheedled his son, "Now, Kevin, do what the doctor says."

The beetle-browed child slunk grudgingly across to the table and clambered up. But that was all he would do. Like many four-year-olds, Kevin resisted every attempt at examination, folding over at the waist or arching his back as necessary to interfere with placement of the stethoscope, tightly sealing his eyes and mouth, clamping his hands over his ears, clutching the edge of the table to resist lying down—protecting himself in every possible way from this unwanted assault. Unlike most four-year-olds who evade an exam this way, he did it with neither whines of protest nor giggles on the edge of tears but with stern glares, peremptory grunts, and then, as I pulled back from my attempts, with a bold, challenging stare and a half-smile that seemed to dare me to try to win this competition. I stared back for a moment, sizing up this little person, then turned to his father and asked him to help Kevin cooperate with the exam.

Mr. Morris looked at me in puzzlement, "What's wrong?"

"I can't examine him if he won't let me. Perhaps you can convince him to. Why don't you come stand up here with us and assure him he's safe?"

"Oh. Sure." He wheezed to his feet and limped the few steps to the exam table, leaning on his cane. "Now, Kevvy, let the doctor do this."

His cajoling tone was now accompanied by a baby-talk lisp. Kevin turned away in a determined pout. I looked pointedly at Mr. Morris, unimpressed by his effort. He grinned and bobbed his head, turned back to Kevin, and barked the child's name. Kevin's head whipped back around, his eyes wide. His body relaxed in defeat. The exam proceeded without difficulty.

As I examined the child, I asked his father whether Kevin's grunting was just a sign of his displeasure at this visit or whether he used words on other occasions.

"Oh, yeah, he talks a blue streak at home. Can't stop that boy from talking. But he don't talk in front of other people. Jimmy—that's his big brother—he was just the same. Never said a word to anybody outside the house till he got to kiddiegarter. And he's just fine now." Another proud paternal grin, shining from those grizzled cheeks, eyes squeezed to slits.

After Kevin and his father left, reassurances about his health accepted gladly, I dug back farther into Kevin's chart. One of my colleagues, some months before, had also been concerned about Kevin's failure to speak— like me, she could elicit no words from him and was leery of the report of his talking "a blue streak" at home—and had referred him to a speech therapist for evaluation. His father, who had been with him on that visit too, had apparently accepted the notion of referral as placidly as he seemed to take everything. However, immediately following that note in the chart was a memorandum, dated several days later. The clinic clerk had called the Morrises to arrange the speech therapy appointment. Kevin's mother had received the call and, according to this note, had become "upset" with the caller. She had angrily denied the need for such a referral and had then threatened to call the county sheriff and her lawyer to charge the clerk with harassment if she were to contact the Morrises again or make any attempt to set up an appointment. The physician who had initiated the consultation had written at the end of the clerk's description of this confrontation that the referral request had been cancelled and that no further attempts at contact would be made. Sounded like a wise decision. I returned the chart and mentally filed away this odd encounter as another in my unwritten anthology of clinic anecdotes.

A few months later, I saw a mother and two-week-old baby who had come to the clinic for the infant's first routine checkup. The student who saw them told me that the mother wanted the formula changed because the baby was spitting up a lot. Usually a parent switches a child's formula without our permission or assistance, but this family was getting their formula through the Special Supplemental Nutrition Program for Women, Infants, and Children (W.I.C.), a chronically underfunded federal program designed to attend to the nutritional needs of impoverished women during pregnancy and of their children through the first year of life. W.I.C. would provide a formula other than the standard, least expensive brand only with an explanatory prescription from a doctor or nurse practitioner. Families often asked us to give such permission, sometimes reasonably, sometimes not. And some of us were tougher than others at needing good "scientific" reasons to justify a formula switch.

Thus I met Mrs. Morris and baby Susie. I did not put this mother-and-child duo together with the father-and-child pair I had met before. Mrs. Morris looked to be forty-five or fifty years old, although I later realized she was only thirty-five then. She was noticeably overweight, thick and stocky, and most of her light-brown hair, streaked with gray, was pulled back into a haphazard ponytail held in place by a rubber band.

As I entered the room she was rocking back and forth in her straight chair, crooning to the baby in her arms.

We had a relatively pleasant conversation. She was a bit abrupt and seemed prepared to argue for what she wanted, but she could not hold back the broad smile that lit her face when I cooed over her baby. Even with the smile, however, she kept flicking her eyes to my face as though she were taking my measure. I had the impression that this was a rather suspicious woman, willing to engage with me up to a point but not granting me any assumptions of benignity. She described the baby's frequent vomiting and told me that her two older children had had similar problems, which had been solved only with the formula change she was requesting. Susie had gained weight well and was clearly a thriving baby; her physical exam was entirely normal. Her vomiting had not harmed her, but I knew and sympathized with how much of a nuisance frequent spitting can be for those who care for an infant. I explained to Mrs. Morris that there was no significant difference, other than the manufacturers' names, between the two formulas we were discussing; that is, there are generally no "scientific" reasons to support switching from one to the other, nothing to lead one to think that a change would take care of a spitting problem, which is rarely caused by formula intolerance anyway. She listened impatiently then interrupted to dismiss my science with her experience.

"All I know is she's got the same problem as my two boys had, and that fixed them, and it'll fix her. She can't handle this milk. She needs the other one. You need to write me for that so I can take it to W.I.C. You people always give me so much trouble up here with getting what I need."

This was her longest speech thus far. I have reproduced it as I understood it. I could not possibly re-create her accent, her idiosyncratic speech that went beyond any regional dialect or impediment that I could recognize. Mrs. Morris spoke like Mrs. Morris, like no one else I have met before or since: an intriguing and often frustrating combination of unique mispronunciations and extraordinarily rapid delivery that made interpretation a challenge and an adventure. There was never enough space within her pressured speech to insert a check on my comprehension, so I just learned to do my best, over the years realizing that everything she said would be reiterated multiple times, giving me ample opportunity to sharpen my translation.

"Okay," I said. "If that's what you're sure works, let's give it a try and see how she does on it."

I was generally in favor of such clinical trials. A month or so on another formula would show who was right with a decisiveness no continuing debate could supply. Moreover, it had not taken me long in pediatrics to learn that, more often than not, the parent was the one who was right in this type of argument; the formula switch usually worked. Why that should be the case in any given situation seemed to me an unsolvable and unimportant question. The goal of pediatric medicine is children who thrive and parents who are happy with their thriving. If it sometimes takes a W.I.C. prescription to meet that goal, so be it.

"I'll write the prescription."

Mrs. Morris looked surprised. I guess she had expected more of a battle. "Okay. Thanks. Go ahead and write it for me now, okay? Make sure you write it like they want you to; I don't want to have to come back here to get another one."

Yes, ma'am.

I wrote while she packed Susie into her stroller for the trip back to the parking lot, and then I watched them wheel down the hall, wondering whether that counted as a good pediatrician-parent encounter.

Two weeks later I saw them again. This time Mr. Morris was with them, and the penny dropped. Of course. Looking at the baby again I could see the striking family resemblances: Susie looked like Kevin, who looked uncannily like their father.

This time the baby was sick. She had lost her appetite and was running a low-grade fever. (She was, however, not vomiting. In fact, I was assured that she had done no spitting up since she had been switched to the new formula.)

Fevers in babies less than two months old are taken very seriously. Their immune defenses are incompletely developed, so they are not as well equipped as even slightly older children to fight off invading microorganisms. Plus, very young infants have a significantly restricted repertoire of symptoms: they may feed poorly, vomit, have diarrhea or constipation, be abnormally sleepy or fussy (or sometimes both), or have a body temperature above or below normal. That's about it. Deciding whether a baby who is fussy and off his or her feed is sick or is just having a bad day (gas? a chafing diaper?) is part of the art of pediatric practice. Attributing fever to a cause likely to be benign, such as an ordinary respiratory virus, is always a leap of faith, not to be undertaken lightly. Given the inadequacies of the immature defense system, a one-month-old infant can go from ambiguous symptoms, that need not imply infection, to being overwhelmed by the infection and unable to be saved, even with the right antibiotics, in a matter of hours. Trusting one's clinical judgment with febrile infants is made more difficult when the parents' observational skills, diligence, and ability to return for medical care as necessary are either unknown or known to be limited; in such situations, watchful waiting is rarely a viable option.

Not only did Susie have a fever, but she looked sick. She was listless, dull, only weakly responsive to stimuli, and had had little to drink all day. Perhaps she was just dehydrated, but we had to be sure this was not a potentially fatal infection. She would have to have an intravenous line placed for fluids and antibiotics, blood drawn for tests, and a lumbar puncture performed to assess cerebrospinal fluid for evidence of meningitis—and she would need to stay in the hospital for at least forty-eight hours, receiving parenteral antibiotics until it was certain that the cultures of her blood and spinal fluid grew no bacteria and that she had returned to normal behavior. Quite a load to hand to any parents of a new baby. I had some passing acquaintance with these parents and wondered how this information would translate within their worldview.

I do not recall what I said to Mr. and Mrs. Morris, only that it took some time to convince them of the potential seriousness of the situation. They were so sure she just had a cold—everyone at home had colds; why not Susie too?—and I had to find a way to say that they could well be right, but the risk to Susie if they were wrong was unacceptable. Step by step, I wrested permission from them, first for blood studies, then for an IV, then for hospitalization. Persuading them to let us do the spinal tap took longest of all, but finally they agreed to everything. Mrs. Morris cried silently—her jaw clenched, tears running down her face—through most of our talking, while Mr. Morris alternated between patting her arm and tugging nervously at his hair (still sticking out around the orange watch cap). I felt for them, so out of their element, being bulldozed by me into acting against their deepest inclinations, albeit for a good cause.

After they had capitulated, Mrs. Morris fixed her teary eyes on me. "You're gonna be in there while they do all this stuff to Susie, aren't you?"

Well, no, I wasn't planning to. I had lots of other patients to see while the residents did the "sepsis workup," a routine set of procedures for pediatric trainees. But, "Yes, I'll be in there as much as I can."

I knew I would have to assure the experienced resident doing the spinal tap that my presence was not intended as interference, but I didn't want to lose the germ of trust—because I had been willing to switch formulas without argument?—between Mrs. Morris and me. Who knows why or how trust forms? We are more used to seeing it in blossom than in seed. Perhaps in these ways, with small proofs of attention and of my trust in her, her confidence in me was being shaped and nurtured.

The workup was completed without difficulty. Mr. Morris went home to see to the boys while his wife stayed behind with the baby. John, a bright and personable fourth-year medical student who was working in the clinic that month to confirm his decision to become a pediatrician, offered to accompany Mrs. Morris to Susie's hospital room. He had been the first to examine Susie this time and at her formula-changing visit two weeks before and thought Mrs. Morris might be glad to have the company of someone she knew, however slightly, as a guide through the unfamiliar corridors of the hospital.

I went to visit Susie the next morning. She looked much perkier—the fluids may have been what she needed after all—but her mother seemed even more haggard than usual after the night beside her daughter's bed. As soon as I walked into the room, she started her rapid-fire talk: Susie is fine, the nurses are crabby and don't change her quickly enough, when can we get out of here, does she really need to stay another whole day, and I need to talk with you about something. I tried to handle each clause separately. She nodded glumly but did not argue when I reiterated why they had to stay at least forty-eight hours.

"And you want to talk with me about something?"

"Yeah, that Chinese student you made come up here with me yesterday."

Chinese student? I wracked my brain. Oh, John, who looks vaguely Asian and told me he has some Filipino blood in his background. "Do you mean John?"

"Yeah, that Chinese man. I don't want him seeing Susie again."

"What's the problem?"

"He tried to touch me. You know. Tried to feel me."

"What?" This was unimaginable. I certainly believed John to be trustworthy, and I knew they had to have been in public elevators and corridors all along the way. What could she mean? "Tell me what happened."

"Well, you know when he first came in to see Susie, you know, a couple o' weeks ago?"

"Yes."

"Well, he kinda picked her up off my lap, you know?"

"Yeah . . . ?"

"Well, the way he sorta took her up, like this." Here she made a deep scooping motion with her right hand, aimed generally at her crotch, and waited for me to finish the thought.

"You mean, you think he was trying to touch you when he did that."

"Oh, yeah. I mean why else would you pick up a baby like that? It's not natural. He didn't have to take her off my lap like that."

"Hmm. Was there anything else? Something that happened yesterday?"

"Yeah, that's what I'm trying to tell you! When we were in the elevator, bringing her up here. I'm carrying Susie and all, and he stands right up by me—in the elevator, with other people there!—and puts his arm around my back and starts patting my shoulder! Like this." She reached her arm around to my far shoulder and tapped it lightly. "Why'd he do something like that?"

"Maybe he thought you needed some support, or comfort? Maybe?"

"Hmmpf. He shouldn'ta done that. It's not right. I don't want to be touched by some Chinese man. I don't know what he was after."

"Gosh, I don't know. John's a very nice man. I'd imagine he was just trying to be kind. Did you say anything to him about it?"

"No! We were on the elevator, I told you! I just got away from him as fast as I could when we got to this floor and told him to go on back downstairs."

"I'm sorry this upset you. Did anything else happen?"

"No, that's all. But I don't want him seeing Susie again."

"Okay. He's only working with us for this month anyway. He'll be gone in a few days. Is there anything else you want me to do about this?"

"No, just that. He shouldn't be seeing little girls."

"Thanks for telling me. I'm sorry it happened. I'll talk to him."

I could not see anything to be gained by arguing with her. I was pretty sure these were her own exuberant fantasies, puzzling and startling (and, yes, irritating) though they were. I felt no need to defend John further, especially because she did not seem to want to take this complaint any further. She seemed satisfied having blurted it all out to me. She was now smiling and eager to talk about Susie's apparent return to health.

Later that day, when the opportunity arose, I took John aside and told him what Mrs. Morris had said. He was horrified—not outraged and indignant, but confused and appalled. I asked for his side of the story, and he described the same actions, but the interpretations were wildly different, as I had expected. Mrs. Morris was going to be someone with whom I would have to be careful, and caution is what I then discussed with John. I assured him that I did not think he had made sexual advances toward Mrs. Morris but that there was definitely something for him to learn from this. John was an easygoing, affectionate man who seemed to enjoy hugging, and being hugged by, the children he saw in clinic and touching them affectionately in other ways—a hand on the shoulder, a pat on the head. I recognized his behaviors because I had been much the same way and had had to learn, as John also needed to learn, to pay attention to limits and to realize that no one—especially a vulnerable child, but also a parent—is fair game for touching.

This is not simply a matter of a newly rigidified atmosphere produced by increasing numbers of "inappropriate touching" accusations. It is much more a matter of honoring a person's bodily territory and not taking advantage of one's position as doctor to invade it thoughtlessly. We physicians cannot assume that our loving gestures will be interpreted as affectionate, as opposed to lustful or controlling, nor that—even if construed as fondness—our affection is wanted by children or their parents. A light touch on the shoulder or arm—a signal of attention and reassurance—is usually all right; it is difficult to misinterpret (although Mrs.

Morris's unpredictable reaction exemplifies the exception) and is some-times essential in particular circumstances to make presence and concern palpable or to make a connection when only a physical link will do. But squeezing a knee, holding a hand, or stroking a head may be unearned and unwanted intimacy. Returning a child's spontaneously offered hug is absolutely okay, even required, and one of the great joys of being a pediatrician. Initiating the hug is another matter. Sometimes it may be the right thing to do; I have certainly given hugs to some adolescent pa-tients, for example, who are struggling mightily and need to know some-one respects their efforts and cares about the outcome. But we should never forget the power differential between doctor and patient (or parent), between adult and child. Who can say no to us?

Children are always at the mercy of other people's needs, perhaps es-pecially their needs for physical contact. There may be nothing quite so comforting at certain times as cuddling a warm, nestling child—and per-haps few things quite so diminishing to a child's sense of self as being made to nestle against his or her wishes, in the face of his or her dislike or fears. Mrs. Morris was almost certainly more mistrustful than most, her reaction to John's gestures radically disproportionate to their intent. But, then again, perhaps she was just uninhibited enough to give voice to what many people, adults and children alike, may feel: "You don't know me well enough, doctor, nor do I care for you enough to make this ges-ture welcome. Step back." Mrs. Morris's over-the-top interpretation of John's actions may have been articulating a deep uneasiness that many of us have about unwanted touch, where sex and power get all mixed up together.

I recall an earlier episode when a male medical student swung his arm around my shoulders and patted me, his professor, while telling me what a great job I had done with the patient we had just seen together. My sense of a breached barrier between student and teacher, my offense at what I took to be his patronizing tone, and, of course, any number of related gender issues fueled my extreme displeasure with his gesture—but I doubt he had a clue that he was received as anything other than a friendly, open-hearted guy. I wonder how often I have been the oblivi-ous, offending toucher.

Susie did well, showed no evidence of bacterial infection, and went home with her parents after two days of intravenous antibiotics. One day soon after she left the hospital, I received a telephone call from a public health nurse in the health department of the county in which the Morrises lived. She had been assigned the task of visiting them to see how their baby was faring. When Susie was a newborn and in our hospital's nursery, astute nurses had assessed the Morris household as a high-risk environment for a baby and had requested a home visit. The request was certainly justifiable; had I been attending in the nursery at that time and first met the Morrises there, I would have put in such a request myself. The home-visit system was designed to be sure that someone was checking up on a newborn when there was reason to believe the baby's caretakers might not be able to care for him or her properly, whether because of financial pressures, social chaos, or physical or mental limitations. Some or all of these conditions seemed to apply in the Morrises' case, so concern was definitely warranted.

The public health nurse was calling not to report her findings from the home visit, as it happened, but to share her consternation. She had called the Morrises to arrange a time for the visit, but Mrs. Morris had refused even to consider it. In fact, beyond simple refusal, Mrs. Morris had announced that anyone who tried to check up on their baby girl would be met at the edge of their property by the elder Morrises, loaded shotguns in hand. The nurse decided not to go.

She then filled me in on what the health department already knew of the family. They had used the department's clinic regularly for free immunizations for the older children but had brusquely and consistently rebuffed all other offerings of assistance. By her account, the Morrises were notorious for their resistance to, even hostile distrust of, the county's various social services. The nurse and I agreed that, as long as they were bringing the children in for care often enough that we could assess their well-being in some fashion, there was not much else to do at this point. There had never been, to her knowledge, evidence of abuse or neglect, just of the depredations of poverty, a lack of education, and a deep-seated suspicion of interfering do-gooders.

I saw the Morrises, in various permutations of parents and children, with some regularity after that and got to know each of them better, but there remained, inevitably, significant gaps in my knowledge. Mr. Morris—James—did not seem to have any steady employment; in fact, I am not sure he did any work, period. The cane was usually present, so I assumed some sort of disability but had no clue what it might be. The description I gave of him at the beginning of this story could be used for any of our encounters as his appearance was remarkably consistent, almost always including the orange watch cap. The oldest child, Jimmy, was fourteen when I began seeing the family, and four-year-old Kevin, newborn Susie, and Mrs. Morris comprised the rest of the household. It was some years into our acquaintance before I began to use Mrs. Morris's given name, Mary. Somehow "Mrs. Morris" just seemed right during the long period it took for us to forge our professional relationship, but she seemed really pleased the day I spontaneously called her "Mary" for the first time. At my request, she occasionally tried calling me "Margaret," but it did not seem to sit well with her. It always came out sounding as though she were trying to get away with something forbidden. I remained "Doctor Mohrmann" or, more accurately, in Mary's compressed speech, "Dar Mome."

Susie never missed a scheduled well-child checkup and came in many other times for complaints usually labeled by her mother as a cold or an ear infection. At first, Mary asked for amoxicillin, the usual antibiotic given for otitis at that time, at virtually every visit. She was not at all pleased when I would not give it to her—Susie had very few ear infections—but gradually she allied herself with me, after a fashion. Her line changed from "She needs that moxillin [her elision]" to "I don't want her to have no medicines she don't need, so don't be givin' her any of that moxillin."

Susie did have occasional discomfort from constipation, and I instructed Mary in how to use small doses of milk of magnesia to help the baby through those troubles. The other over-the-counter medication I introduced her to was the liquid form of the anti-inflammatory drug ibuprofen. This I recommended for fever and the irritability of teething, and I told her the appropriate dosing regimen. Soon Mary was "doctoring"—her term—Susie with great assurance, entirely convinced of the broad-spectrum efficacy of these two medications. She would call to tell me that Susie had the "flu" again, but that she had things under control.

In a tone that defied objection or modification, she informed me that she mixed a little milk of magnesia and a little liquid ibuprofen in the cap of the milk of magnesia bottle and gave that to Susie every four hours or so. Worked like a charm, she assured me. I am a pragmatic pediatrician; what works, as long as it does not bear risk of harm, is generally fine with me.

"Okay, but don't use any container bigger than that bottle cap, and no more often than every four hours."

"Sure," she would huff in reply. "I know that! It's only the flu!"

I soon learned that "flu" was the label Mary gave to virtually all sickness, especially respiratory afflictions, but also gastrointestinal upsets. When the time came that she began telling me of her own illnesses, I found that "flu" also applied to any combination of the headaches, dizziness, and malaise that came to characterize Mary's own struggles with obesity, diabetes, hypertension, and ever-present stress.

I could not have known at the start that Mrs. Morris's phone calls, initially to report on the baby's "flu" episodes—or bowel problems or teething—and her own doctoring efforts were to become the dominant motif of my relationship with her. As Susie got older and I saw more of the boys in clinic, she would call about their health issues too. Then she started phoning to talk about problems the boys had in school. Later it became her troubles with her neighbors and various county authorities or with the truck or with Mr. Morris or with her own health. There were weeks when she would call almost every day, sometimes three or four times a day. Then there might be a month or two with no contact—the misleading eye of the storm—before the calls would start up again for another run.

At first, Mary would call the clinic to talk with me. If I were not available, she yelled at the clerk who gave her that news, haranguing, demanding that the clerk find me, that someone else talk to her—no, not a resident, not a nurse!—that the hospital stop calling her (who did that?), that they not mail stuff to her. She was almost always loud and sounded angry, her speech unsettling in its rapidity and near incomprehensibility. I would hear about these disturbing calls in detail the next time I was in clinic. The reports were relayed with exasperation or outrage, of the "I don't have to put up with that woman" variety, and with the implicit, sometimes explicit, message that I was responsible, if not for her behavior at least for controlling it. Mrs. Morris had quickly become identified as "mine," and I often found myself apologizing for her anger or their distress. I tried to help the clerks find ways to respond, including recommending that they tell her forthrightly that her tirades were unacceptable and would not be tolerated, but few had the courage, even over the phone, to face her down. I gave Mary that message directly more than once, but each time I did she insisted that she had been dealt with rudely and disrespectfully and was merely responding in kind.

Eventually I convinced her to call not the clinic but my office when she needed to talk with me. I had at that time an extraordinarily good secretary, Kathy, who could accept Mary in all her oddness, talk gently but authoritatively with her, and assure her that I would get her messages. I promised Mary that I would always call her back if I were not available when she called and tried to stick to that pledge, although sometimes it was *very* hard to call her back. I remember well the first time I called and got her answering machine. The first thing I heard was Mary's voice yelling "Don't hang up!" I was so startled, I immediately and obediently responded, "I won't!" Then I realized that her voice, in an only slightly calmer tone, was now telling me that she could not come to the phone, but I had *better* leave a message. She was not about to tolerate any hangups or any unidentified callers on her phone.

Interspersed among the telephone calls were numerous clinic visits. Many of these were scheduled appointments, but some were spontaneous appearances: I would step out of an examining room and see the Morrises at the end of the clinic hall, advancing on me. "There she is! C'mon, James!" Mary would be pushing Susie in her stroller, James a bit behind her, dragging Kevin by the hand while the boy tried to pull away, whining for the toys in the waiting room. Or, bent over my paperwork in the residents' room, I would hear a loud, hoarse attempt at a whisper, calling my name. "Dar Mome! Hey, Dar Mome! I need to talk to you!" And there at the door would be Mary, beckoning me to a huddled conference in the hallway. My colleagues studiously ignored these forays by the Morrises but later, when I returned from handling the latest question or demand, would find a way to remind me how pleased they were that the family belonged to me and not to them.

The face-to-face encounters provided the connecting sparks that forged my relationship with Mrs. Morris. I learned to tell how things were going from her facial expressions and how well she was groomed—when she was pleased with her life, she looked fifteen years younger—and to treasure the uncommon sweetness of her broad smiles of delight and affection, when her china-blue eyes would gleam and hold my gaze in a moment of shared pleasure in Susie's development or of mutual amusement at some absurdity in the latest of her outrageous tales. Such moments led me to care deeply about her and her family, helped me handle the more difficult times, especially the strident, fragmented demands that came so often over the phone. It is also true that the cumulative hours I spent listening to the broken pieces of her life transmitted over the telephone wires prepared me to recognize and cherish the times of untroubled joy when they came.

Initially, I dreaded her calls. Actually, to be honest, I never stopped dreading them. I did, however, stop resisting them, and that relaxation went a long way toward defusing my trepidation. The calls were long, loud, jangling cries for help that I could not possibly give, pleas to fix the unfixable. No doctor I know likes being presented with an incurable problem, an unresolvable question: I did not like it. My frustration made me abrupt, at times dismissive. But, after a time, when I knew beyond doubt that the calls were going to keep coming and I was going to have to answer them, my technique—as much a mode of self-preservation as attentive medical care—became merely to listen. I set aside, with more or less success, my ingrained doctor's sense that my job was to fix things, accepted my inability to do that, and just took the calls. That method was not too difficult to pull off; Mary spoke with such rapidity and vehemence that there was not much for me to say anyway, not much breathing space in which to insert remarks.

Occasionally, in the midst of her saga, Mary would ask, "So, what can you do about this?" and then pause for an answer. I found that if I said in return something like "Gee, this must be really hard for you" or drew a connection between this episode and some other issue in her family's life, she would start talking again, apparently not noticing that I had not answered her question. After twenty or thirty minutes of this, she would abruptly say, "Okay, thanks a lot. Bye," then hang up. Many were the times I sat staring at the dead receiver, wondering what had just happened. After a time, I began to understand that this was why she called: to be heard, to articulate, as well as she could, her chaotic life and have someone pay attention, carry the burden with her, and agree that it was hard. Mary, in her inimitably demanding, wearing fashion, had forced me to become the doctor *she* wanted for herself as well as for her children.

As an aside, it is perhaps my experiences with the Morrises that most clearly illustrate that, for most of my career in academic medical practice, I was the recipient of a gift not available to all doctors: time. I had time to listen to Mary Morris on the telephone, just as I had time, when running the P.I.C.U., for extended conversations or periods of pregnant silence, for accompanying children and parents as they explored the dangerous territory at the border of life or the threshold of death. This luxury of time was one of the benefits of being a salaried faculty physician whose income was not directly dependent on how many patients were seen in a day and whose compensable activities were agreed to include time spent teaching, conferring, and researching.

I would argue, of course, that adequate time for taking care of patients (and oneself, for that matter) should in no way be regarded as an extravagance, but as a necessary resource for good doctoring. Regrettably, ever-worsening financial constraints on medicine, among other factors, have reduced the essential element of time to nothing less than a luxury, generally unattainable. Were I in practice today, it would be considerably more difficult to find the time to listen to Mrs. Morris day after day, to learn what I needed to know about Jermaine Rogers' parents' beliefs, to respond to Jennie Daugherty's adolescent crises. Having said that, however, I must also make a counterargument: we all find the time to do what we consider to be important and claim insufficient time for those activities we find, not unimportant perhaps, but less necessary, less compelling. I gave listening to, accompanying, and waiting for my patients and their parents a high priority; these tasks of attending drew me in ways that reading journals, not to mention doing paperwork, never could. I expect that this would still be true were I in practice today, but also that the pull of the increasing volume and urgency of paperwork would greatly intensify the conflicts over time already inherent in the profession of medicine.

After Mary decided to bring Susie to see me regularly, I also started seeing the boys, Kevin for checkups and the recurring "flu," Jimmy less often for occasional aches and pains. A year or two into this routine, Mary and I had a couple of odd conversations about my role in their lives. She insisted that she wanted Susie to have a "woman doctor":

"Because Susie's a girl and all, you know, and I think it's a good thing for a girl to have a woman doctor. But James, he don't think the boys oughta be going to a woman doctor, you know. It's okay with me, but James, you know, he just thinks it ain't right. He thinks you're fine for Susie, I mean he likes you and all, but the boys need a man doctor, don't you think?"

"Well," I mumbled, taken aback, "not necessarily, but I'm happy to set them up with a 'man doctor' if that's what you want."

"You know, you're nice and all, and Susie likes you, but woman doctors just aren't as good as man doctors, you know, don't you think?"

At this I laughed out loud. "Do you really expect me to agree with that? I *am* a woman doctor. Of course I think woman doctors are every bit as good as man doctors." Still chuckling, shaking my head.

She laughed a little too, tentatively, not sure what the laughter was about. "Well, you know what I mean, I just think man doctors are better, so it's okay for you to be Susie's doctor, but we want Kevin and Jimmy to have a man doctor."

We had this conversation two or three times. Each time, she slandered "woman doctors"—and, not incidentally, her daughter, worth only a second-rate physician—apparently without the slightest notion that it might be an inappropriate thing to say in a conversation with me, Susie's "woman doctor." Each time, I laughed a little more and found my affection for this strange and clueless woman growing. She never said any of this angrily or haughtily, but rather as though she were having a discussion about the weather and what "everyone knows" about it. She *knew* man doctors were better, so of course I must know that too. Oddly enough, I felt warmed to think that she had reached such a level of trust that she could talk with me so guilelessly and accept my amused disagreement. I could not *argue* the subject with her; argument would have been pointless, like trying to convince her that snow was not cold. She knew better. Plus, by the time we had our last chat on this subject, it had become clear that it was all talk. Nothing had changed. I had arranged for one of our male pediatric residents, supervised by a male faculty member, to take over care of the boys, but Mary continued to insist that their appointments be with me. Finally, she called me one day about one of the boys' needing to be checked for something or other.

"So, does this mean I'm still the boys' doctor?" I asked.

"Sure," she said, puzzlement in her voice. "You're the children's doctor, all of them."

"I thought James wanted the boys to have a man doctor."

"James," she snorted dismissively. "I say you're their doctor, you're their doctor."

Fine with me.

As this pediatrician-parent relationship took its peculiar shape, molded especially by the recurring phone calls, I began to appreciate what I was learning about their lives and about my role as their pediatrician. The calls, while no less intrusive and exhausting, became privileged communications from a world I could scarcely imagine. It had not taken long for me to recognize symptoms of mental disorder in Mary—the pressured speech, the deep suspiciousness that went far beyond the stereotypical wariness of a rural person in the face of citified professionals, the too-easily accessed anger—but I tried to keep myself from thinking of her in diagnostic terms. Seeing the events of her life through her eyes was an education in itself, about both the nature of the Morrises' existence and the particular perspective that Mary's uniquely skewed vision offered. Moreover, each call, with its set of demands and expectations, compelled me to think again about my obligations and limitations, as both a doctor and a human being.

From pieces of information gathered through years of phone conversations, I formed a composite picture of the Morris family's life. Mary and James had married when she was in her early twenties; she became pregnant with Jimmy a year or so later. (They had not had premarital intercourse, she told me sternly and spontaneously when Jimmy, at the age of eighteen or so, moved in with his girlfriend, much to her distress.) After their marriage, they lived for a year or two with her mother, who eventually decided that she could not stand having James around, so they moved out on their own into the house they still occupy.

Their property, located about forty miles from the clinic in a rural county, has been in James's family at least since the 1930s. The house and the surrounding few acres seem to be the only real asset the Morrises have. The house has electricity but no running water. There is an ancient wringer washer on the back porch for which Mary has to haul water. Kevin's inevitable wringer injury to his arm, fortunately not severe, was the first one seen in our clinic in many years, wringer washers having become obsolete decades before. According to Mary, she was constantly cleaning house, fending off the dirt that her husband and sons tracked in, careless of her housekeeping. When she was not scrubbing floors, carrying water, or washing clothes or dishes, she was cooking or tending to the children in some fashion. As a rule, in each call Mary inserted an account of the housework and errands she had accomplished before using the telephone. Although she rarely complained about James, she dropped enough hints for me to gather that he did next to nothing around the house, by her estimation, and rarely took responsibility for the children.

Mary's neighbors and their activities seemed to play an inordinate and uniformly negative role in her existence. One next-door neighbor in particular, in Mary's view, was engaged in a perpetual vendetta against the Morrises and, specifically, against Mary. At one clinic visit, Mary told a complex and bizarre tale of a message left on her answering machine by this woman, a message Mary interpreted as a semipornographic invitation to Mary to enter into a sexual relationship with the woman. Mary talked at length about how disgusting the idea was to her, how offensive the invitation, how malicious the neighbor. I wondered if, like the earlier episode with John, this was an instance of Mary's sexual fantasies overtaking her perception of innocent events. This neighbor—or perhaps another, I was never quite sure—at various times reportedly sabotaged the Morrises' truck, killed their dogs, pulled up plants in Mary's garden, left "anonymous" threatening messages on their phone, called the sheriff on them, tried to kill Kevin (the means used were not clear), tried to burn down the Morrises' house, wanted to buy the house and land to make them move away, or were themselves moving to get away from the Morrises.

I had no way of knowing whether any of the tales were factual. In most cases, I assumed they were extreme overinterpretations of upsetting or even ordinary, if not wholly imaginary, happenings. Because Mary's routine and immediate remedy when she felt threatened was "Call the sheriff!" I usually did not have to decide whether the threats sounded real enough (Is someone really trying to kill Kevin?) to recommend such a step. More than once, I wondered what it would be like to hear the sheriff's perspective on the conflicts he was called to adjudicate in Mary's neighborhood, but I settled, though not easily, for my role as Mary's credulous sounding board. It seemed more important that she know she could come to me with these tales and be heard—even sympathized with for the obvious distress she was suffering, no matter its source, so that I could maintain my position, however limited, of overseeing the children's health.

But, of course, even the children's welfare, not to mention my role in it, was often difficult to fathom in the midst of the ongoing chaos described to me over the phone and sometimes in person. Jimmy, as he careened through adolescence, dropped out of school and did a lot of near-suicidal things with alcohol and dirt bikes. By the time he was eighteen, the bones of his legs and jaw had been pinned and wired back together a couple of times, he was working as an unskilled laborer on construction sites, and he was living in a trailer with a girlfriend his mother despised. This summarizes almost four years of intermittent telephoned pleas to me to fix him, the school, his surgeons, his boss, or "that girl." I examined Jimmy several times because of psychosomatic symptoms that kept him from the misery of attending a school where he was convinced he would not succeed and where he was ridiculed as a "stupid hillbilly." I negotiated the terms of his release from academic prison with school administrators. Later, I wrote letters to his boss, asking for the time off he needed to keep follow-up appointments for his many dirt bike injuries. But mostly I listened, hearing Mary struggle with Jimmy's growing pains and, especially, with the unwelcome recognition that at eighteen he had become an adult she could no longer coerce into going to physical therapy against his will, much less into moving back home.

At about the time Jimmy moved out for good and his tribulations could be safely shunted to a back burner, Kevin became the focus of concern. Now eight years old and in third grade, Kevin had already amassed a lengthy record of disciplinary actions at school, including several suspensions for fighting with classmates and talking back to teachers. Now he was in much bigger trouble after an episode in which he—innocently in Mary's eyes, but malevolently and threateningly by the teacher's account—had "waggled his penis" at his female teacher when she chased him down to the boys' bathroom after he had run out of her classroom. For months, Mary called with new iterations of the story, always demanding that I somehow fix this problem, whose consequences had grown from Kevin's immediate suspension from school to his placement in a special school for troubled children. My one consistent offering, that Kevin have a thorough psychological evaluation and, if indicated, some form of therapy for his disruptive and self-defeating behavior—a recommendation I had been pushing for at least two years—was, as always, rejected. Nevertheless, she kept calling, spilling out her concern and dismay, her fears and anger in ever-more frenzied formulations of the situation and its portents.

Then one day Mary's call was more jumbled than usual, her demands for my aid more frantic. The ultimate result of Kevin's apparently sexual threat toward his teacher was a serious investigation of the Morris family by the county's office for child protection. A court date had already been set at which a judge would determine if Kevin and Susie should be taken away from their parents. While I understood without difficulty the county's position, I also knew how devoted Mary—and James too, in his own laconic way—were to their children. I had wrestled time and again, during my relationship with the Morrises, with the question that haunts all pediatricians in the face of certain families: when do their aberrant ways of living, their odd perspectives on the world, their reclusiveness, their lack of interest in education and worldly success—all the troubling and "abnormal" characteristics of a family like the Morrises—add up to an environment that is dangerous or damaging enough to justify tearing apart family bonds?

Evidence of physical harm, or its realistic threat, is a relatively clear-cut motive for taking children away from dangerous parents. In contrast, what is one to do about the shiftlessness of a father like James, the manifest "craziness" of a mother like Mary, or parental ineffectiveness or unconcern in the face of their children's behaviors or attitudes that endanger themselves, their futures, or other people? What combination or degree of these parenting deficiencies rises to the level of justification required to sever family ties and abrogate the rights of parents to rear their children as they see fit? I do not have the answers to those questions, but they are questions that I, like my fellow pediatricians, have struggled with in any number of situations.

My own conclusion to the dilemma, always tentative but also always reconfirmed in this case, was that, chaotic as their household surely was, the Morrises' devotion to their children and constant attention to their welfare as they understood it outweighed my concerns. There were never any signs or suggestions of physical abuse and, although one can never know what goes on behind the closed doors of a family's house, I believed Mary to be a person who would neither resort to violence with her children nor allow anyone else, including James, to do so. I performed the physical examinations of the children required by the investigation and found, as I expected, no evidence of recent or past abuse, nor could I glean any hint of inappropriate sexual behavior from private interviews with each child.

One of the bizarre aspects of the case against the Morrises was that, according to Mary, it had been initiated not only by the school but also by Jimmy, who was asking to have custody of his younger brother and sister. Mary, not surprisingly, was reeling with hurt, anger, and terror at the thought of losing Susie and Kevin and at Jimmy's treason. I reeled too, not knowing whether her information was accurate, whether there had been horrors in their family life driving Jimmy's quest of which I was ignorant, or whether Jimmy was in any way capable of caring for his siblings. I still do not know the answers, but the conclusion of the trial judge was that the children should stay with their parents and that Kevin had to have a thorough psychological evaluation as well as psychotherapy, if that were determined to be necessary. Mary was all for it, finally.

By the time I left clinical practice, Jimmy seemed a figure of the past, although Mary still mourned his absence from their home. Kevin was behaving relatively well in a much more controlled school environment, although his psychologist had already abandoned his futile efforts to accomplish any sort of therapy with Kevin and his parents. Susie was, by all reports, thriving in kindergarten and seemed the healthiest of the lot thus far, although, as she cocked her head, squinted at me, and smiled a sort of crafty half-smile, I wondered whether her uncanny resemblance to Kevin was more than skin deep. Social service officials came by to visit their home periodically. Mary allowed these visits grudgingly—I got a call after each one to hear her baffled outrage—having realized from the terror of the court case that her previous modes of defense against such intruders could cost her her children.

People often ask me, now that I am no longer in the practice of pediatrics, whether I miss it. I answer them truthfully: no. My present work is so satisfying and so much a natural outgrowth of those years of doctoring that the transition has been seamless, and I have no significant sense of loss. But that is not entirely true; I do miss Mary. Troubling, intrusive, frustrating as she was, she had wormed her way into my heart, my conscience, and my perception of myself as a physician. The only guilt I have felt about leaving practice has been guilt at taking away from Mary her one attentive listener. It is not immodesty on my part to say that I doubt she will find another. There are many other good listeners in the practice of medicine, but for some reason Mary and I had forged a particularly rich bond of respect and trust that may not be reproducible.

I remember a day some two years into our relationship, after a long stretch of innumerable exhausting phone calls about some string of crises, when I was seriously questioning my ability to continue working with her. I was sitting in the residents' room of the clinic, jumping each time the phone rang, praying it would not be her again, when she materialized at the door beside my desk, pushing toddler Susie in her stroller. I got up slowly, guardedly, to see what she wanted. Mary ducked her head shyly and then, with a sweet smile, thrust into my hands a bouquet of flowers.

"They're from my garden, you know," she said. "And Susie, well, she wanted you to have them because she really likes having you as her doctor. And we just wanted to say thank you for all the good things you've done for us and for being the children's doctor and all."

A couple of years later, at the end of a visit in mid-December, on her way out of the examining room door with four-year-old Susie, Mary abruptly pushed into my hands a plastic grocery bag. In it was a $2.99 box of chocolates (the price tag was still on the box). "Susie saw this in the store and wanted to give you something to say Merry Christmas," Mary said gruffly, but unable to suppress her smile of pleasure at giving me something. Susie looked pleased too, and I thanked her warmly, but I understood that the gift was from Mary.

Flowers and candy were not the only gifts Mary gave me. She embellished and expanded my understanding of the vocation of physician that had begun forming in my experiences during residency, my realization that the practice of medicine asks far more of us as human beings than simply our cognitive expertise or our ability to prescribe the right medications and perform skillfully the correct procedures. Mary asked not just for my knowledge but for me. She called me to respond to her as one human being responds, in love and compassion, to another human being who is in trouble and suffering, and specifically to respond by letting her describe to me her life, otherwise unimaginable. More than anyone else in my practice, Mary taught me about the "waiting" part of attending. Our relationship happened on her terms, in her timing, not mine. She placed the phone calls; my job was to wait for her call, to wait to hear what she had to say, to wait for her to articulate the pain and distress, to wait for the mysteries of her life to become clearer, the unknown parts of the story to take their places in the narrative. I learned not to push ahead with questions, the answers to which, even were they forthcoming, I would not be able to fathom if I did not wait long enough to know her and her life sufficiently well.

When I closed my practice, in addition to talking with Mary about my departure, I wrote her a letter, explaining the change and giving her the name of my faculty colleague who would now be the children's pediatrician. A few weeks later, I got a letter from her in response. I reproduce it here as she wrote it; the original is laboriously scrawled on lined paper torn from a spiral-bound notebook:

Dear Dr Mohrman
    I got your letter
you dont want to be a doctor.
Dr. _____ kids doctor now. I miss you from being kids doctor. Kevin is doing great in school. he really miss Jimmy bad. Jimmy move out. Because of woman in back have trobles with. We all miss him want him to come back. But he wont. Susie she in kindgarden she turn five this month. Love school. go every day. Susie + Kevin say miss you as there Doctor.

Say tell you Hello. You as a great Doctor. I want to say thank for your help with kids all three even big kids thanks for great ear of listen to my probly. its hard to find Doctor like you. Writeing to let you know I am thinking of you. and great person you are. Write to me some time let me know how you doing. if you come back to office let me know kids allway need Doctor like you.

Love Mary Morris + family

Three months after I had moved on to my new position within the university, Mary found me once again. Early one morning, she, James, Kevin, and Susie, in an uncanny replay of all those times they had sought me out in clinic, appeared outside my new office door. She needed to talk about Jimmy's latest escapade and what I was going to do about it.

Chapter 14

Against All Odds

MY FIRST MEMORIES of Janet Walsh come from the time when she was nine years old and in the fourth grade. She came to the clinic with some regularity, at times accompanied by her mother, other times by her maternal grandmother. Almost all the visits were for some sort of ache or pain normally acquired in the life of a nine-year-old, never portending anything major. With each encounter I was struck by two unforgettable things about Janet: her size and her spirit. She was an unusually tall and significantly overweight child, and she evinced a sort of hearty defensiveness that was startling in a girl of her age. Her ashy blond hair was usually pulled back tightly into a ponytail or two pigtails, which accentuated the plumpness of her rosy cheeks and punctuated each toss of her head with an affirming flip. Janet seemed always ready to fight, ready to toss off any feeling, inquiry, or gesture directed toward her that smacked of sentiment or gentleness. She had an air about her that proclaimed, "I'm just fine, thank you very much, and don't ask further." Even at nine.

The most memorable of those fourth-grade visits was one of my earliest encounters with her mother, Brenda (Ms. Walsh insisted, from our first meeting, on being called by her first name only; I do not remember that she ever used my name, in any form). The family resemblance, physical and spiritual, was marked. I do not recall the reason for this particular meeting, but I do remember once again bringing up Janet's weight and the need to put some controls on it, if not to reduce it, at least to keep it from increasing quite so rapidly. We had a separate clinic, with its own expert physician, specifically focused on matters of weight, and I offered a referral to that doctor for evaluation and guidance of Janet's eating and exercise habits. My concerns were blown off by both Janet and her mother, and their folie à deux was blatant.

Brenda looked at Janet with a sly smile and said, "Well, we have to keep her in fighting trim, don't we?"

"I'm sorry. I don't understand."

Janet and Brenda laughed together in delighted knowledge and conspiracy. Janet began the explanation: "The boys in my class, they're always betting each other whether they can beat me in a fight. But they never can!"

"So," her mother chimed in, "we can't let her get any smaller if she's gonna keep winning!" This said with a look of maternal satisfaction, as though we were discussing her child's skill in academics or music rather than her role as the standard of manhood for fourth-grade boys.

"Oh. . . . How often does this happen, Janet?"

"Pretty much every day," she said, tossing her head with tentatively defiant pride.

"So," Brenda turned serious now, "we don't have any interest in her losing any weight. She's just fine as she is. I want her to be able to defend herself."

Once again I launched into my explanation about present and future health risks.

Brenda cut in sharply, "Yeah, I know you doctors say that kinda stuff. You've always gotta make out that something's wrong. Well, Janet's just fine. Forget it. Come on, Janet. We don't need to stay here any longer."

As would often be the case with this pair, the visit ended abruptly with Brenda marching out the door and Janet hanging back long enough to wave good-bye and smile before turning to catch up with her mother, who was steaming ahead toward the elevator. I shook my head in confusion, as I often did after these visits. What just happened? And what was I, the pediatrician, called on to do, if anything, about an obese nine-year-old girl who, encouraged by her proud mother, had adopted the role of class tough? More to the point, what *could* I do that either of them would hear or accept?

Soon after that, Janet began coming to the clinic only with her grandmother. I did not see her mother at all for a few years. I got an explanation from her grandmother one day while Janet was busy elsewhere (I do not recall why, but certainly not having blood drawn; that was not something Janet allowed) and eventually pieced the story together with bits I learned from Janet: Brenda had a long-term live-in boarder-cum-boyfriend named Art, described by the grandmother as a shiftless alcoholic. Janet despised him. They fought constantly, mostly about Art's hogging the TV and the most comfortable chair in front of it and, to a lesser extent, about his never helping around the house but demanding service from Janet of the "bring me a beer, kid" variety. Janet and her grandmother, together and separately, laughed scornfully at my queries about whether Art had ever sexually molested or threatened Janet. Their consensus seemed to be that he was not capable. This child, who would take no guff from a fourth-grade boy, was not about to be bossed around by a slug like Art, and because Brenda, consistent with her usual construal of mothering, had no intention of asking Art to leave, Janet had to go. Thus the decision that all would be better if Janet lived with her grandmother for a short time. Brenda and her mother lived within several blocks of each other, so Janet still saw Brenda regularly but was now primarily cared for by her grandmother. The "short time" turned into almost three years.

The other, equally difficult part of the story was that Janet's grandmother was suffering from A.I.D.S. and trying to deal simultaneously with her prognosis, her declining health, and her stubborn and willful granddaughter. Apples not falling far from the tree, Janet's grandmother's personality was not too different from that of Janet and her mother: prickly, defensive, and closed. No amount of sympathetic inquiry from me elicited any details from her about her situation, short of an agreement that it was all very hard, yes, but we manage. Pride plus distrust of medicine in general—perhaps of me in particular, except that they kept coming back and asking for me—combined to form a formidable obstacle to my comprehension and, at times I feared, to Janet's care.

During this period, I continued to talk about Janet's weight, which was increasing apace, and was met with much the same resistance. Stories of fourth-grade prowess faded away, but denial of the problem remained strong. Janet's grandmother said Janet was just "big-boned," as she certainly was, and that she was carrying the right amount of weight for her size, an irrefutable circular argument. Stymied on the weight front, I began pushing another possibility—counseling. It seemed an obvious need: the chaos in her mother's household, life with her slowly dying granny, a persistent problem with school avoidance (fortunately handled with steely determination by her grandmother, who really wanted Janet out of the house and at school every day). But, no. No one in that family, I was assured, had the least interest in seeing anyone even vaguely involved with "mental health." Janet was not crazy, and I needed to stop suggesting she was. All my protestations to the contrary, that this had nothing to do with being "crazy," were futile. I could do no better than settle for a wary truce. I would bring up the subject from time to time, and they would toss it back at me in a pointless game.

It was during this time, as Janet got a bit older, that she seemed to become more attached to me and began to talk more freely with me. I would take her with me, out of the examining room to retrieve some needed implement or check her eyesight or some such, in order to have some time alone with her, away from her grandmother's resistance to discussions of any sort. From Janet I learned a piece of information that made sense of a lot of what I had seen: Brenda was bipolar and took her medications only irregularly. When she was on them, things were relatively stable, although her personality was still hostile and demanding. When she was not taking them . . . well, it was better for Janet to live with her grandmother.

Janet, old beyond her years at eleven, was the only child in this extreme family. She had turned her body into a sturdy defensive wall, keeping herself well padded and projecting no hint of physical fragility. She had also erected an equally thick psychological barrier that enabled her to face her chaotic world with a disconcerting combination of nonchalance and bristling hostility. No one would mess with Janet, was the clear message. And no one would get close either. Except sometimes she was just an eleven-year-old girl with too much to carry. Sometimes she would cry as she talked with me about her grandmother's illness and how much she did not want to go back to living with Brenda and Art, or about how difficult school had become.

Now that the worth of her classmates had to do with their attractiveness to each other rather than their ability to face the biggest kid in class in a duel, Janet was lost. There was a boy in her class she really liked, but he ridiculed her for her size as much as the rest of her classmates did. All she knew to do was fight back; her gentler emotions had never been honored. On several of our visits during those years, I spent a lot of the time listening and holding her, cradling this large, dear child in my arms while she cried. During this time, the symptoms that brought her to clinic became less the aches and pains of combat and more the vaguer, subtler signs of heartache, anxiety, and loss. She complained of lightheadedness, recurrent headaches, and morning nausea that would assault her at the school bus stop, only to disappear shortly after she resigned herself to being at school yet another day.

Shortly before she turned twelve, Janet moved back in with her mother and the ever-present, unchanged Art. Her grandmother had become too sick, too weak to deal with Janet's needs; her respite, such as it was, was over. Things seemed to go well for a while, which probably meant that Brenda was taking her medication. They worked out ways in which Janet's contact with Art and potential flash points could be held to a minimum. But it was not long before Brenda's basic inability to care for Janet came to the fore, and Janet's needs were once again ignored. The anxiety symptoms and school avoidance became worse. Janet was in a terrible bind. She hated going to school, where she had not yet assembled a persona acceptable to her peers. She hated being home, where the insufferable Art held sway and arguments with Brenda were the daily news. Her schoolwork suffered, of course, even though she was an innately bright child; she missed many days and could not work at home, she reported. She was bright enough not to fail a grade, but her marks never reflected her abilities, as she well knew. Brenda was unconcerned and, generally, unavailable.

On one visit, shortly after her return to her mother's house, Janet played one of her characteristic games with me, refusing to talk about the physical complaint for which she had asked to see me. Brenda became furious with her, said she was wasting her time, and stalked out of the clinic—all the way out, leaving Janet there alone with us. As Brenda stormed out of the room, Janet suddenly looked bereft, even panicky, but only momentarily before switching back to her familiar shrug-and-sneer defense. But then, with Brenda's angry presence out of the room, she opened up about the reason she had come to clinic, we had one of our better visits, and I made sure she had bus fare to get home (they always came to clinic on the city bus, a system with which Janet was very familiar).

This situation struggled on for about a year, with Janet showing up in the clinic at least every couple of weeks with her usual complaints, with or without Brenda. Mostly she would just check in with us—not only with me but with the clerks and nurses who had let her know that they also cared about her. She felt at home with us, I think, at least to whatever extent Janet could be at home anywhere.

And then, one day, shortly before she turned thirteen, she came to clinic on a day I was not there. She was accompanied by her aunt, Brenda's sister Louise, who figured ambivalently in Janet's life. Louise, an elementary school teacher, was one of the only stable influences within Janet's family, but she also made a lot of demands—often more angry than loving, to hear Janet tell it—that Janet pull herself out of the chaos she lived in, chiefly by performing well in school. I was delighted that Janet had someone asking that of her, but chagrined that the expectations were not accompanied by the emotional support Janet so badly needed.

On this day, Louise brought her to the clinic because she had learned that Janet had had sexual intercourse for the first time the night before. Mark, a man in his thirties on parole from prison, had been staying in the Walshes' house at Brenda's invitation and sleeping with Brenda. (Art still lived there too, but by this time had his own room, with its own TV, and was slipping further into the alcoholic haze in which he would die several years later, having shrunk into a relatively innocuous presence in the house.) The night before, while Brenda was away, Mark had seduced Janet. As Janet told the examining physician, she had sort of wanted it; she did not fight him, but it was not so good—it hurt—and the next morning she was pretty scared and sorry she had done it. She called Louise, who brought her to us.

Fortunately, the physician attending in clinic that afternoon was our adolescent specialist, expert in matters of child sexual abuse and especially adept at helping a violated child talk about and deal with the event. Given Janet's age, there was no question that a crime had been committed. The police were called; Mark was arrested and returned to jail to await trial. Janet, being Janet, refused a pelvic examination and the blood tests necessary to screen her for human immunodeficiency virus (H.I.V.) and other sexually transmitted diseases (S.T.D.s). She was given an appointment to see me the next week.

On that return visit, Brenda accompanied her. A furious Brenda: furious with Janet for having sex with Mark, furious with interfering Louise for bringing Janet to the clinic, furious with us for calling the police so that Mark was now "out of my bed and back in jail for nothing!" She was furious with everyone except "poor Mark," wronged by an idiotic legal system. Brenda did not think Janet lied about what Mark had done; she believed they had had intercourse. She just did not see why we thought it was such a big deal, or why we thought it was Mark's fault and not Janet's.

I knew Brenda well enough not to try reasoning with her, plus I was too angry with her entirely misplaced loyalty to make the attempt. I said, "That's the law. Janet's not old enough to give consent, not old enough to know what she's consenting to. She's still young enough to need the protection of the law *and* her mother." The last sentence I added with some heat, knowing full well that Brenda would either ignore me or leave the room in response. She ignored me. I went on to argue for the necessity of testing Janet for H.I.V. No way. Janet adamantly refused to be "stuck." Brenda refused to consider it a valid risk:

"I'd know if Mark had H.I.V. Don't you think I'd know it? My own mother had it. He doesn't have it."

I explained, to no avail, that you cannot know by looking if someone has H.I.V., that a person can carry the virus for years before showing any signs of A.I.D.S. I may as well have been talking to the chair. Brenda pulled out her typical argument: "You doctors are all alike, always looking for something to do to people that you can make a little money off of. It's a waste of time, and we're not doing it." With one last "Forget it!" Brenda slammed out of the room and, as before, left the clinic entirely—which gave me the chance to talk with Janet alone, something Brenda would not allow when I had asked earlier.

Although Janet would still not agree to H.I.V. testing, she did talk more about what had happened. She felt terrible about it, but that feeling was now mixed with guilt that she was the reason Mark was back in jail.

I told her that Mark had put himself back in jail and that she was in no way responsible for that, but my words made little apparent impression. She had felt too responsible for too much for too long to imagine this too had not been her doing. Besides, she had wanted it too, had wanted to know what it was like. She even confessed that she was afraid no one would ever want her that way. So, when Mark did, how could she say no? If she had known it would cause so much trouble, maybe . . . but she had not known that, had not known he was committing a crime. And, she added, with that stubborn glint back in her eye, there was no way she would accept the legal definition of "age of consent" as having anything to do with her. Of course, she was old enough to say yes or no.

I asked her then how things were at home with her mother. Pretty bad, apparently. Brenda frequently and loudly blamed Janet for Mark's reimprisonment and, perhaps more to the point, for Brenda's having lost her sex partner. I could not fathom her mother's apparent indifference to what seemed to me the salient issue: Mark had had sex with twelve-year-old Janet. Even if Brenda could not muster enough maternal feeling to care about the injury to Janet, was she not at least jealous? Was she not bothered that the one night she was out of the house Mark not only found another sex partner but chose Brenda's own daughter? Apparently not. Mark was entirely exonerated of being anything other than "natural," to use Brenda's label for his crime. As Janet talked about her mother's anger and blame, the tears came. Then she told me what hurt the most: Brenda was going regularly to visit Mark in jail. Janet did not want to see him ever again, but her mother was making every effort to take care of him, while doing nothing to take care of her own child. Janet's baffled pain was palpable—and unfixable.

I saw little of Janet over the next several months, only heard from others who were there how difficult it had been for her to testify against Mark at his trial. But testify she did, as did a friend of hers, also twelve and also raped by him. Mark would now be in prison for a long time. Janet's years of learning to defend herself, to present herself to the world with strength and a readiness to take the offense saw her through that ordeal, as it saw her through life at home with her mother.

Janet took to hanging out downtown with a group of disaffected teenagers given to hackysack and marijuana. Each time I saw her, her hair was a different color. She seemed to revel in feeling a part of this group and paid as much heed to my warnings about tobacco and pot as she had to my concerns about her weight, which, from my perspective, was as much a problem as ever. She told me proudly of her boyfriend(s), but denied having sexual intercourse—she said her experience with Mark had convinced her to stay away from sex for a long time—and bragged about the cool things she and her friends did.

School was not one of the cool things. An eighth-grader now, she was still limping through on borderline grades, missing as many days as she could get by with. She continued to come to the clinic periodically with complaints of morning dysphoria, even an occasional "faint" at the bus stop, wanting medical excuses for school and, perhaps, explanation and resolution of the symptoms. Brenda accompanied her on most of these visits. Since Mark's trial, Brenda had been oddly subdued, almost pleasant in her interactions with me. I figured she was taking her medications again. The old Brenda was still there, however; several times within the same encounter she would bounce between certainty that Janet's symptoms were a ploy to avoid school and insistence that we find out what was wrong and fix it. Agreeing with her about the school avoidance did nothing to quell her demands for a diagnosis and a remedy in order to relieve her (Brenda) of this problem, but any offer to test for alternative diagnoses would be shot down immediately with her "you doctors are all alike" refrain.

At one point, Janet had an episode that sounded suspiciously like a seizure. I was not at all sure this was part of her usual malingering but could not convince Brenda to let us do an electroencephalogram. She did not want any tests, and, besides, she was not about to have Janet labeled as epileptic. She knew what it was like to be branded with a mental illness—I could not convince her of the distinction between psychiatric and neurologic disorders—and it was not going to happen to Janet. What she did agree to was a visit to a neurologist for a second opinion about Janet's symptoms. When she called the number I gave her to arrange the appointment, the clerk answering the phone identified the place as the "epilepsy clinic." Brenda hung up on her and called me in a fury. No amount of explanation that going to an "epilepsy clinic" is not tantamount to a diagnosis of epilepsy—that that is where the pediatric neurologist sees patients—could shake her. Fortunately, the symptoms that triggered my concern did not recur, and I became increasingly sure that they were part of Janet's generalized symptoms of anxiety and, perhaps, depression.

When Janet entered high school in the ninth grade, she started doing much better in her schoolwork for a while. I was delighted for her and asked what she thought was making the difference. She told me that her aunt Louise had promised to help her with college if she would keep her grades up. Finally, a positive influence—someone telling Janet she is worth supporting! However, midway through the fall semester she and her mother came in for a clinic visit to have fourteen-year-old Janet tested for pregnancy. Far from being worried about the possibility, the two of them were giggling together in a way I had not seen since their consensus about Janet's status as fourth-grade punching bag. Janet had a set of baby clothes with her that they thought were just the cutest things ever and wanted me to admire. (When I reflected on this visit later, I had a sudden, detailed recollection of the clinic visit with Crystal twenty years before when she, full of longing and glowing with hope, also brought baby clothes to show me.)

It was scarcely worth asking the standard question, "What will you do if you are pregnant?" But I did and got the expected answer with the expected affect: they looked at me as if I were an alien life-form and said, almost in unison, "Keep it, of course." Duh.

I got Brenda out of the room—she was surprisingly accommodating—so I could talk with Janet alone. She said she had decided a few months before to start having sex with this newest boyfriend, whom she liked a lot. When I asked about her previous resolve to abstain after her experience with Mark, she blew that off as a decision made by her younger, less mature self.

"I'm ready now. I want it. Besides, having a baby would be so cool."

"What will happen to school?"

"Oh, I'll go back." Then, with one of those "How dumb are you, anyway?" looks, "Of course I'm going to finish school!"

"Who'll look after the baby while you're at school?"

"Mom will."

I gently reminded Janet of some salient features of her mother's maternal abilities.

She stuck out her stubborn chin and said, "Well, sometimes the baby can stay with my boyfriend's mother, and Mom's not so bad right now. She's really excited about this. She wants me to have a baby."

In the midst of our conversation, the pregnancy test came back negative. Relief made my knees weak. I sat down as I read the sheet, then told Janet that she was not pregnant.

"Oh, shoot!" she said. "Oh, well, I'll just save these"—here she started folding the baby clothes—"for another time. Maybe it's too early for me anyway. It was gonna be hard, with school and all. Still . . . Mom's gonna be disappointed."

She was as lighthearted and unconcerned as I had perhaps ever seen her, as blasé as she had been before the test report came back. I started talking with her then about birth control, about preventing pregnancy—and S.T.D.s—but she barely listened as she patted the little pile of colorful togs.

"No," she said, "those pills make you gain weight. And it's not right, you know. If I'm supposed to get pregnant, I'll get pregnant. So, can I go now?"

"Let me get your mother in here to tell her too, okay?" I said, hoping against hope that I could raise the matter of birth control to better effect with Brenda.

Brenda's response to the negative pregnancy test, much like Janet's, was an easy acceptance. Neither relief nor depression, just a sort of "Oh, well, we can always try again" reaction. I began telling her that I had been talking with Janet about birth control, but she stopped me abruptly with a hand up like a traffic cop: "No way. I don't want her on those things. They're terrible for you. If it's time for her to have a baby, she'll have a baby."

In the face of their fatalism, I could only say, "If you change your mind, let me know. Having a baby will really mess up your school plans, and"—I had to say it—"it's just not fair to give a baby a fourteen-year-old mother."

Brenda snorted and rolled her eyes. Janet said blithely, "I could do it. Even if I am only fourteen."

They gathered their things and walked out, ambling down the hall arm in arm, a sight I had never seen in the five years I had known them. Finally something had brought them together; the folie à deux had returned with a vengeance.

Janet came in to see me only occasionally over the next several months, usually for help with her acne or relief of a sinus infection. She had reverted to her previous poor school performance, but this time it looked as though she would not be passed to the next grade, a prospect of little concern to her, except for its potential to delay her final freedom from school. She researched information about the earliest age at which she could legally stop attending school, all the while assuring me, with her usual aplomb, that she would get her G.E.D. (General Equivalency Diploma) if she did not finish high school. School was "stupid," as far as she was concerned, and especially trying was the insistence that she participate in a physical education class, which asked of her physical feats she claimed she could not and doubtless would not perform. Each of the many times she asked for a medical excuse to get out of gym I refused, telling her she needed gym more than almost anything else she was doing. "Whatever," became her resigned response.

At about the time the next school year was to start, one of the residents working in the pediatric clinic told me about having seen Janet in clinic a few days before. This time she *was* pregnant. The resident said Janet, now fifteen years old, seemed not only very happy about it but also very serious about doing everything correctly for the welfare of her baby. She had agreed to a referral to the Teen Health Center (T.H.C.), where she would be followed closely and counseled well throughout the pregnancy. I spared a thought for Janet's choice to come to clinic when she knew I would not be there, and I thought I probably understood that decision.

Shortly thereafter, I received a phone call from the social worker at the T.H.C., who wanted to talk with me about Janet, newly enrolled as one of their prenatal patients. Janet had given permission for the social worker to get any necessary medical information from me, but what she wanted more was some handle on how to understand Janet. She was impressed with her determination to do everything recommended for her and to be a good mother for this baby. Janet had already agreed to participate in parenting classes and, later, in a developmentally enriched day-care program for the baby that would ease her return to school. The program included after-school assistance to the mothers—help with both baby care and schoolwork—and Janet seemed very willing to be part of it. I explained to the social worker as well as I could Janet's nature, something of her difficult home situation, and a lot about her personality: the prickly and the soft sides, the ways I had learned to talk with her so she would listen, how important it was to her that her opinions be respected and that she be regarded as fully competent, mature, and capable of shouldering almost any burden.

In turn, the social worker told me not only about Janet's attitude toward the pregnancy but also about the baby's father, Damon, who was sixteen and doing about as well in school as Janet. He had yet to come to any of her prenatal visits, but Janet insisted that he was closely involved and intended to be around to help rear their child. As the social worker told me this, I could picture the determination in Janet's face and the steely glint that would tell Damon that he would, by all means, be involved, or else. Janet could still be the standard of manhood.

I saw Janet a couple of times during her pregnancy, when she needed treatment for the sinus infections that plagued her from time to time. She was as content and as determined as I had ever seen her. I also kept up with her through the staff at the T.H.C. She was faithful in her visits and compliant with the recommended regimen. She continued in school during most of the pregnancy but did not do particularly well. Aunt Louise had angrily withdrawn her promises of support when she learned of Janet's pregnancy, but the promises had come too late anyway and with too much baggage.

In May of the year Janet would have been completing tenth grade—she was now just shy of sixteen—her daughter was born. The labor was long and the delivery perilous for Janet; she lost a great deal of blood and required several transfusions. The baby was initially thought to have an infection and needed intravenous antibiotics and close observation for the first few days of life. I got a call from the nursery to let me know of her birth and to discuss their concern about Janet's insistence on taking the baby home before the doctors thought she should be discharged.

Someone on the staff knew of my relationship with Janet and thought I could help. Right, I thought wryly. Like Janet listens to me. But I went.

Janet was in the nursery, swathed in a gown, sitting in a rocking chair by the baby's bed, and holding her daughter in her arms. She beamed when she saw me, and I was captivated by the sight of this often so angry or sullen child now wreathed in smiles as she adored her own daughter. Captivated and wary. I knew Janet too well.

I decided to play ignorant visitor without an agenda, so I cooed over the baby—a beautiful girl with a full head of soft black hair—and let Janet tell me of her adventures with delivery and now with the baby. Her daughter was named Le-André, an amalgam Janet had spent months concocting, stirring it round until it sounded right. She was already referring to her as "Lee." It became clear as she talked that Janet was quite willing to go along with what the nursery doctors wanted to do but that Damon, the baby's father, was insisting that the baby was all right and, in odd echoes of Brenda's habitual charge, that the doctors were just doing what doctors always do to make more money. As Janet said that, she stole a look at me and we started laughing. Then, while I listened to her think through this conflict out loud, Janet came to her own conclusion that Damon was "just throwing his weight around to prove he's the daddy. Well, he's the daddy all right, but I'm her mother, and what I say goes. She's staying here until they say she can go." For once, I was grateful for Janet's stubbornness and her need to let no one else take control—and grateful that Damon had made himself and not the doctor the one whose attempt to take charge had to be countered.

I asked Janet where they intended to take the baby for pediatric care. I had hoped they would come to me and said as much. I wanted to work with Janet through this new part of her life too.

She said, "Well, I wanted to bring her to see you, of course. I told Damon you've been my doctor all these years, and I wanted you to be Lee's doctor too. But he's got this idea that she has to have a private pediatrician, somebody in town. He doesn't like the university. That's part of his problem. He wanted her to be born at Martha Jeff [the local community hospital]. He thinks the university doctors just experiment on people and don't take care of them. Of course, I know that's not true, so I said I was going to have the baby here, period. But I think I'm going to have to give in to him on this one. She's his baby too."

I had to admire the maturity of this compromise position; this was a new, improved Janet. I was impressed by her understanding of Damon's reasoning, her wish to care for him, her willingness to bend in places. I also knew that the pediatrician Damon had chosen was an excellent doctor. I told her I thought their choice was just fine, that Lee would be in excellent hands. I also assured her that my door was always open, if she had a question or concern, wanted a second opinion, or just wanted to talk. I left her with a hug and found the nursery doctor to tell him the baby would stay as long as necessary—and I was honest enough not to take credit for that outcome.

About a month later, on my clinic list for the afternoon, there was Lee's name. She was to be seen for a diaper rash. Lee looked great, clean, beautifully dressed; the rash was easily handled. Janet looked good too, happy and proud. She was very comfortable with the baby, showering affection on her, careful of her and attentive to her needs. She was being a good mom. I told her so, and she smiled broadly at the praise. Then I asked her why she had brought Lee to see me instead of her pediatrician. She mumbled something about not being able to get an appointment with the other doctor. I pushed her a little, and she admitted that she had just wanted to bring Lee to me. The other doctor was very nice, but he was not me. She knew me and trusted me and just could not see taking Lee anywhere else. She had talked to Damon about it, and he had fussed but finally given up. I confessed my pleasure at her choice. We arranged for Lee's next regular well-child checkup, at two months of age, and I asked her to get Damon to come with them so he could meet me—and I could check him out.

All went well for the first several months of Lee's life. She thrived, growing and developing normally, happy and cooing each time I saw her, always clean and well dressed, and very well cared for. Initially Janet was flourishing too. She was so proud of Lee and increasingly confident in her ability to care for her properly. Damon was living with Janet in the Walshes' house because Janet wanted him to share in the parental duties. He and Brenda did not get along well, and Janet often had to mediate between them, but she professed herself used to it all and not particularly bothered by it. Art stayed in his room watching TV all day and was little more than a placeholder in the house. He acknowledged the existence of the baby and Damon, but showed little interest in either.

Janet and I talked about school starting back in the fall. She had everything arranged: Brenda would baby-sit sometimes, Damon's mother sometimes, and for much of the afternoon Lee—and Janet, when she got off school—would be at the program for teen mothers that the T.H.C. had found for her. She professed herself ready to return to school. She was not happy about leaving the baby all day, but she was determined to do well in school. As she said, "Now it's not just me. I've got Lee to think about, and she's not gonna have a high school dropout mother. I need to go to college to make a good life for us, and I'm gonna do it." Louise was back in the picture, charmed by the baby and once again offering Janet support dependent on successful work in school.

Janet's first semester back was a combination of ninth- and tenth-grade courses, making up for what she had failed before and what she had missed during the later stages of her pregnancy. She threw herself into her schoolwork, determined to do well—except for gym, a class she still could not make herself attend. Unfortunately, she needed it in order to graduate. I talked with the school counselor about working out a gym-equivalent that Janet could pass and was gratified by the school's level of commitment to her success and willingness to work something out. That semester Janet made all A's in her academic courses. I was astounded. I had known that she was bright but had not imagined she could perform at that level.

Janet was quite proud of those grades, but tired and uncertain if she could keep up the pace it took to make them. She told me what her life was like. Each morning she showered and dressed, then got Lee ready for the day—bath, dress, feeding, instructions for Brenda or whoever was to be the caretaker that day. On to school for a full day, the late afternoon spent in parenting classes and study hall at the day-care program with Lee. Then she came home to prepare dinner for the household; Brenda refused to cook, saying it was Janet's responsibility now, especially with Damon in the house. After dinner she cleaned up, put the baby to bed, and did homework until she fell asleep herself, only to be wakened off and on through the night by Lee. Damon refused to get up with the baby during the night, claiming ignorance and ineptness. He also did nothing to help around the house; when he was there, he watched TV and fought with Brenda. He played with Lee occasionally, but did nothing to take care of her, not even diaper changes. Brenda, although she was more likely than Damon to spend time with Lee, also brought her back to Janet when she cried or needed changing.

Janet was in a fix. Aunt Louise had offered to take Lee for an occasional night, and Janet was just about ready to let her. Not only was she complaining about sleep loss, but she was also beginning to reflect on how her life had narrowed down. She missed being out with her friends. An edge of resentment at always being tied to the baby crept into her voice, focused not on Lee but on Brenda and Damon.

We talked about whether it was helpful to have Damon in the house, seeing that he contributed nothing and was the reason Brenda used for her nonparticipation in the housework and preparation of meals. Janet had a string of reasons why she could not ask Damon to leave, although she had clearly thought about it more than once. There was no longer a place for him at his mother's house; she wanted Lee to grow up with her daddy around (Janet's own father was known, but never present). The primary reason seemed to be Janet's need to continue believing that Damon loved her and wanted to be with her. I said no more, other than supporting her need to take care of herself and encouraging her to let Louise help her.

When Janet came in for Lee's nine-month visit, I asked her how things were going. She looked exhausted. School was terrible; her grades had plummeted, and Louise was angry with her again. "I kicked Damon out," she said flatly.

I put my hand on her arm. "What happened, Janet?"

Damon had dropped out of school months before. Janet had insisted that he get a job if he was not going to school and, after considerable prodding, he did get some kind of work. She expected him to contribute money to the running of the household, but he always claimed he had nothing left after his own expenses. Janet eventually became suspicious and contacted his boss, only to find that Damon was being paid well and regularly, much more than he had told her. Then she found a couple of Damon's friends and interrogated them. Damon had been spending his money on another girl and drugs. It was not clear which sin infuriated her more. Drug use was the reason she gave for kicking him out, insisting that she would not put herself and her child in that peril: "If they come after him for drugs, and they know he's living with me, they'll take Lee away from me. That's not going to happen. I told him to get out right then. He's gone."

I asked her how she felt about it, and her defiant chin came up: "Good riddance!"

"What about his seeing this other girl?" I pushed gently.

Her chin looked slightly less defiant and trembled a little. The other woman was an old girlfriend whom Damon had promised Janet he had nothing to do with anymore. But it turned out that he had been seeing her all along, even while Janet was pregnant. He was using Janet for free room and board—and, Janet insisted, "Because he really loves Lee. She's the apple of his eye."

A few months later, Janet let Damon back into her life briefly, after he begged and made big promises; the reconciliation lasted less than a month. During the time he was back with her, she was arrested for fighting in the street with his other girlfriend, who, Janet claimed, ambushed her and pulled a knife on her. Janet was unscathed except for a few bruises, the charge was dropped when the other girl failed to appear on the court date, and Damon was out on his ear again.

In the midst of this escalation of chaos, Janet's desire to live more like a carefree teenager surfaced to stay. She told me about evenings when, after she put Lee down for the night, she went out with her friends, staying out until early morning, trusting Brenda to listen for the baby's cries in the night. One morning she had found Lee standing in her crib, screaming, Brenda nowhere to be found. Janet's hard-earned maturity, which knew that Brenda could not be trusted, that her own first responsibility was to her baby, was at constant war with her adolescent urges to be carefree and put responsibilities off on "adults," no matter their record. We talked long and hard about this problem, about my obligation as Lee's pediatrician to see that she was being adequately cared for. I told her forthrightly that I might be legally required to call her caseworker to investigate the possibility of neglect. Janet was furious at that but quickly lapsed into despair: how was she going to have any time for herself, any fun? I asked about Louise's offers to keep Lee occasionally overnight. Janet's ambivalence toward her aunt was a barrier. She wanted to take Louise up on her offer, but she knew it would come with a lot of unwanted, resented advice—demands, really—about how she should be living her life, taking care of Lee, and so on. A high price to pay, indeed. But, as I pointed out, she might have no alternative if she wanted an occasional break from being a mom.

Several weeks later, I received my first phone call from Louise. She and her husband were now happily caring for Lee most weekends and some weeknights. They thought it would be best if Lee stayed with them permanently, with, of course, entirely liberal visiting privileges for Janet. Didn't I think that was a good idea? After all, I knew what Janet was like, not to mention Brenda's instability. Janet was too young to have full responsibility for a child, and, besides, she needed to focus on her schooling.

I let Louise talk and eventually heard what was behind this call and her proposal. Louise and her husband had wanted children of their own, but for some reason had never conceived. Lee was like a gift; she was perfect for them. They wanted to adopt her (although they would be sure to remind her that Janet was her real mommy) and give her everything she needed. They had stable incomes and a nice house in the country with a big yard, away from all those bad influences in and around Brenda's house.

"What does Janet think of all this?" I asked, not believing Janet would entertain the idea for a moment.

"Well," she said, "we haven't talked with her about it yet. We wanted to run it by you first."

"I don't imagine Janet will agree to this."

"Yes, well, we thought that, if she didn't agree, you would be willing to testify that it would be in Lee's interests to live with us instead."

Ah, now I see. . . . "Actually, I think Janet's trying very hard to be a good mother for Lee, and she obviously adores her. I can certainly see that it's good for Lee to spend time with you—good for Lee and good for Janet—but I can't agree that Janet should not be her mother anymore. That would be too cruel to Janet and there's no basis for recommending it. I would testify on Janet's behalf, not against her."

Unlike her sister Brenda, Louise did not respond in rage. She sounded more deflated—and surprised. "Do you really think Janet can be a good mother for her?"

"By what I've seen, she *is* a good mother for Lee. She pays attention to Lee's needs. Just look at the fact that she brings her out to stay with you. She's not perfect, by any means, and she has a lot to work through, but none of it would be helped by taking Lee away from her."

"Oh, well, we didn't really want to take Lee away from her. . . ."

"But that's what it would mean, wouldn't it? You know she won't agree to it without taking it to court. And I don't think you can win in court. You'll just make sure that she'll never let you see Lee again. I don't think this is a good idea."

Soon after that, I saw Janet, and she told me that Louise was becoming "a real bitch" about Lee. She was not going to leave Lee with her anymore because Louise kept saying things like, "One day you'll come to pick her up and we won't be here. We'll just take her far away where you won't find us." So much for Louise's being the stable one in the family.

Janet said, "I told her, 'If you lay one hand on this baby, if you do anything to try to take her away from me, I'll kill you.'"

The next thing I knew, Janet and Louise had patched things up, and Louise was keeping Lee occasionally again. When I asked Janet why she had decided to trust Louise again, she said matter-of-factly, "Because she knows I'd kill her, that's why."

Louise called me again to give me her version of the current situation. She and her husband had agreed that it was just too much stress in their lives to even think about fighting Janet for the baby. They would just enjoy their time with Lee and try to keep Janet's trust so they could still see the baby sometimes.

Janet dropped out of school somewhere along the way. I do not remember at what point; it had for so long seemed inevitable. She got a job bagging at a grocery store, insisting in her usual resolute mode that she would get her G.E.D. Lee continued to thrive, and Janet continued to dote on her and to leave her with Louise when she needed a night out. The last few times I saw Janet in the clinic, she seemed happier and surer of herself, still saying that Lee was the best thing that had ever happened to her. She and Brenda had reached a sort of amicable truce; they lived in the same house, but saw little of each other. By mutual agreement, Brenda rarely baby-sat for Lee.

Janet's last visit to me came shortly before her eighteenth birthday. She came, this time without Lee, for a physical exam because, she told me proudly, she was signing up with the Job Corps. She would have to live in another town, about an hour away, for at least a year of training and would be able to finish her G.E.D. there. Lee was going to stay with Louise while she was gone; they had reached a very clear agreement about what that did and did not mean. Janet would be able to see her most weekends. She was excited about her future in a way I had not seen before.

I reminded her that this was our last visit, that I was leaving clinical practice. She had not forgotten and thought it was a neat coincidence that we were both going off to change our lives at the same time. Yes, neat. I told her how good it had been for me to know her all these years, what a good person and what a good mother for Lee I thought she was. She smiled broadly and thanked me for taking care of her and Lee, for being there. We had a long hug, and I left her with tears in my eyes. So long, Janet, farewell. Good luck, brave girl.

Epilogue: Still Attending

I still don't know what to say, I don't even know what to write,
because there's too much to say and write and because I know
both too much and too little about it.

—Martin Winckler, *The Case of Doctor Sachs*

As I was completing this book, I wrote to Mickey's parents, Mary
and Marshall Madary. I wanted permission to use their names, but, more
than that, reliving the story had made me want to talk with them, see
them again. I had remained in contact with the family for some years
after Mickey's death, but, as people do, we had lost touch; our last contact had come with news of Chris's marriage in 1983. They called when
they got my letter, and we arranged a time for me to visit. We began
catching up on the phone: they told me of their move to a condominium
apartment after retirement, their teenaged granddaughter, and where
Chris, Joey (now Joe), and Jenny are now and what they are doing.

Driving the few hours from my home in Charlottesville to theirs outside Baltimore, I wondered what this reunion would be like. They had
asked me to bring the draft of my chapter about Mickey, and I expected
reading it would be painful for them—writing it had certainly been so
for me. What would we talk about? Would the story be okay? Would
our memories of that time be troubling, or widely divergent?

It was wonderful to see them again—still so recognizably, quintessen-
tially the Mary and Marshall I had met almost thirty years before: embracing, welcoming, comfortable to be with. Their condo is filled with
framed photographs from the past twenty years of the children and their
families. In their bedroom are two earlier pictures of the children, taken

when Mickey was about four and eight years old. A large photograph on the wall beside the guest bedroom is a portrait of the family in 1978, taken, Marshall told me, at Chris's insistence: "He really wanted a family picture, so here it is." One bookcase is filled with photograph albums, carefully organized by Marshall after he retired; Mary pulled one out to show the snapshot of me in my Halloween getup in Mickey's hospital room—the same photo I have.

We talked for hours, through dinner and a late-night slice of cake Mary had made, and for more hours the next morning, over the brunch she fixed before I drove back home. Mickey entered the conversation sporadically, almost glancingly, mirroring the way she inhabits their lives (our lives, I should say)—always there, as reference and touchstone, never forgotten, a real part of the continuing saga, but not a mournful preoccupation.

The talk was about their family. More than once they told me that they had heard—from the oncologist, the social worker, and others— that a crisis like Mickey's illness and death will either break a family apart or bind it together for good. They know, without question, that they are in the latter category, and they know also that the futures of their surviving children were irrevocably molded by the events of 1974. The family seems exceptionally and happily close-knit, secure within a bond sustained by frequent telephone conversations and holidays and vacations spent together.

Most of the stories I heard that did not concern travel adventures were about illnesses and doctors. There have been other family members, adults, with leukemia. With each diagnosis, the extended family has remembered Mickey and reached out to protect Mary and Marshall from reliving her illness: "This isn't like Mickey. They can do more now." There have been difficult encounters with brusque and tactless doctors; some are stories of breathtaking arrogance and insensitivity. Recounting those experiences led them to remember a few of Mickey's doctors about whom Mary can still say "I hated him!" There have also been memorably good interactions with physicians that, in the telling, called forth different, more pleasant episodes from Mickey's hospitalizations. It is clear, and not surprising, that their perspective on the events I recount in chapter 4 has definitively shaped their reception of and reaction to later encounters with illness, dying, and the medical profession.

They had a lot to tell me, bringing me up-to-date on important parts of their lives together, compressing twenty years of history into several hours' narration. It was good to be at another intersection with them, letting our lives cross at a different but not unrelated point, receiving their stories again. They are well and whole, happy in their rich family life.

I prefaced their reading of Mickey's chapter with anxious apologies about the vagaries of memory and warnings about the pain of returning to those dark months, and I admitted my trepidation at their reading the story written from my perspective: "You know, it's inevitably really about me more than anything." They brushed off my concerns and assured me they were prepared for whatever was in it. They read it after I left for home. The next day Mary e-mailed me. Among other things, she said, "We both read the chapter. . . . I will tell you that it brought back a lot of things that I forgot about, and I guess it's a good thing that we can forget. We can forget things (not Mickey), but bad things that happened to her and to us also. It seems to get a little easier with time."

Like the others whose stories I tell here, the Madarys are, and will be, still healing. And I am, and shall be, still attending.

Notes

Introduction

1. Frank acknowledges anthropologist Julia Cruickshank as his source for the "think with stories" idea and phrasing. Arthur W. Frank, *The Wounded Storyteller: Body, Illness, and Ethics* (Chicago: Univ. of Chicago Press, 1995), 23–24.

2. In this effort, I have been fortunate to have as a model Kate Scannell's insightful book of stories from her practice, *Death of the Good Doctor* (San Francisco: Cleis Press, 1999), in which she has expressed, in her own lucid and compelling voice, what I hope also to display in my work: a constant faithfulness to the patient's experience, as observed by a witness permanently changed by what she has seen.

3. Anne Hunsaker Hawkins, "Medical Ethics and the Epiphanic Dimension of Narrative," in *Stories and Their Limits: Narrative Approaches to Bioethics*, ed. Hilde Lindemann Nelson, 168 (New York: Routledge). Professor Hawkins's splendid and moving book, *A Small, Good Thing: Stories of Children with HIV and Those Who Care for Them* (2000), is another welcome model of thinking with stories.

4. See Jack Coulehan and Anne Hunsaker Hawkins, "Keeping Faith: Ethics and the Physician-Writer," *Annals of Internal Medicine* 139, no. 4 (2003): 307–11. The essay is an excellent, thought-provoking guide for the doctor who writes about her or his patients. Both the essay and additional discussion with Professor Hawkins have pushed me to make my moral deliberations and decisions as transparent as I can.

5. For more on this distinction, see the explanations provided in John Stratton Hawley, *Saints and Virtues* (Berkeley: Univ. of California Press, 1987), both in the editor's introduction (at xiii–xv) and in Peter Brown, "The Saint as Exemplar in Late Antiquity," in *Saints and Virtues*, ed. John Stratton Hawley (Berkeley: Univ. of California Press, 1987), 5.

6. John Lantos, pediatrician and ethicist, has passionately delineated the distinctions between the technical skills of medicine and the human skills of good doctoring in his provocative book *Do We Still Need Doctors?* (New York: Routledge, 1997) and in a more narrowly focused essay, "RVUs Blues: How Should Docs Get Paid?" *The Hastings Center Report* 33, no. 3 (2003): 37–45.

7. These examples of two types of conversion are more memorably, and succinctly, presented by Gerard Manley Hopkins, *The Poems of Gerard Manley Hopkins*, 4th ed, ed. W. H. Gardner and N. H. Mackenzie (London: Oxford Univ. Press, 1967), 54, in his poem "The Wreck of the Deutschland": "Whether at once, as once at a crash Paul, / Or as Austin [Augustine], a lingering-out sweet skill."

8. "Child Life" is an established profession whose practitioners—most holding college or graduate degrees in the field—attend specifically to the psychological, social, emotional, and educational needs of children in hospitals. By helping children keep up with their schoolwork, engaging them in forms of play that address their inexpressible fears, providing safe havens in the playrooms of countless hospital wards, these dedicated care providers can transform a child's illness experience.

Chapter 9

1. *Hemodialysis* is accomplished by direct filtration of blood obtained from an artery, usually in the arm. The blood circulates through a filtering machine and is then returned to the body through a vein, often in the same arm. In most cases, the process requires several hours beside the machine, three or four times a week; for our pediatric patients, it usually meant an overnight hospital stay each time. *Peritoneal dialysis*, in contrast, occurs within the patient's abdominal cavity. Fluid is instilled into the cavity via a large catheter stitched to the overlying skin, and blood is filtered across the peritoneum, the capillary-rich membrane that covers the abdominal organs. Some hours later, the fluid is drained and replaced with fresh fluid, so that the process goes on continuously. Patients and/or their parents can be taught the procedures so that peritoneal dialysis can be accomplished at home and even at school, without taking the children away from family, friends, and study.

Chapter 11

1. Jermaine's parents are African Americans. I am indebted to Mildred Best, a chaplain at our university hospital, for enlightening me about a characteristic aspect of many African Americans' Christian faith, which she elucidates as "the belief that God is a *Waymaker* who can make a way out of no way. In the context of terminal illness this belief can translate to 'When the doctor says no, God can say yes.' " See Mildred Best, "African American Spirituality Perspectives and End-of-Life Care," *Bioethics Matters, A Newsletter for the Friends of the Center for Biomedical Ethics* 10, no. 4 (2002): 1.

D1004192 28043